Praise fo~ ~~~~~~~~ *Minds*

"*Wounded Minds* sho ～～～～～～～～～～～ ~cially by the leaders of today's a~ ～～～～～～～～～ in military suicides and some～ ～～～～～～～ nd benefits conclude thi～ ～～～～～～～ ～nd Atty. Birnes a our g~ ～～～～～～～ ～ots on the Ground.'"

—James Squires, M.D., was a Flight Surgeon for Strategic Air Command during Vietnam, as well as a state Senator, and founding President of the Endowment for Health

"The book offers practical solutions for proper diagnoses and treatment and discusses reforms necessary in systems that play a role in creating the problem and then deny responsibility for the problem. The authors explain how an instinctual protective response instead turns into, for some, an unrelenting problem that affects one's basic ability to work to level."

—William C. Holliday, MD, PS, is a Police Psychiatrist specializing in Posttraumatic Stress Disorder. He is psychiatric consultant to major police departments in Washington State and full spectrum of federal law enforcement agencies

"Once again, the authors delve into the human brain in order to help the public understand the psyche of others. This time, the focus is on the warriors of this great nation, the American veteran. As a veteran of the United States Marine Corps and the son of a Marine Corps Vietnam veteran, this book helps all of us understand the complex mind of the combat veteran. I recommend this book to all who proudly served this country and those who want to fully understand the difficulty of Post-Traumatic Stress Disorder and other combat related conditions."

—Detective Kenneth L. Mains, Founder and President,
The American Investigative Society of Cold Cases (AISOCC)

"Dr. John Liebert has provided a meaningful and incisive service to veterans and our country with his significant research to heighten public awareness by identification of the invisible wounds of war which increase the risk of the lethal outcomes. Medical practitioners, government officials, military personnel, and families all need to read this provocative book which identifies the inner struggles of our veterans returning from combat situations. Dr. Liebert suggests action needs to be taken. We would all be well advised to review his findings and seriously consider his recommendations to address this critical issue to protect the veteran and the people within his or her sphere of contact."

—Charles C. Mulcahy, USAF retired, former Chair,
Milwaukee County War Memorial Center
and advocate for enhancement of the rights of veterans

Wounded Minds

Understanding and Solving the Growing Menace of Post-Traumatic Stress Disorder

John Liebert, MD, and William J. Birnes, PhD, JD

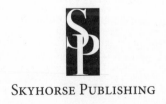

SKYHORSE PUBLISHING

Skyhorse Publishing books may be purchased in bulk at special discounts for sales promotion, corporate gifts, fund-raising, or educational purposes. Special editions can also be created to specifications. For details, contact the Special Sales Department, Skyhorse Publishing, 307 West 36th Street, 11th Floor, New York, NY 10018 or info@skyhorsepublishing.com.

Skyhorse® and Skyhorse Publishing® are registered trademarks of Skyhorse Publishing, Inc.®, a Delaware corporation.

Visit our website at www.skyhorsepublishing.com.

10 9 8 7 6 5 4 3 2 1

Library of Congress Cataloging-in-Publication Data is available on file.

ISBN: 978-1-63450-287-0
Ebook ISBN: 978-1-5107-1366-6

Printed in the United States of America

CONTENTS

Foreword by
Mike Masterson

One of the most important trends in policing over the last few decades has been the growth of "community policing" and its relationships with specific constituencies or vulnerable populations within the community for whom the motto "to preserve and protect" has special importance. Those special populations look to the police, the most visible form of government, to provide leadership in their communities and to better serve and protect them. One of the most promising and certainly deserving practices that helps achieve this is to better serve military veterans in crisis. Recent wars in Iraq and Afghanistan have resulted in many soldiers returning to communities with internal conflicts continuing to rage on emotionally, mentally, and even physically. When these conflicts become too much to bear, the results are often tragic, including suicide and aggression against others—sometimes resulting in police intervention.

According to statistics from the Substance Abuse and Mental Health Services Administration (SAMHSA):

- Almost 18.5 percent of service members returning from Iraq or Afghanistan have Post-Traumatic Stress Disorder (PTSD) or depression, and 19.5 percent report experiencing a traumatic brain injury (TBI) during deployment.
- In 2008, 47 percent of all current Department of Defense (DOD) service personnel were binge drinkers.
- Nearly 50 percent of service members who need treatment for mental health conditions seek it, but only slightly more than half who receive treatment receive adequate care.
- In 2010, the U.S. Army's suicide rate among active-duty soldiers dropped slightly (162 in 2009; 156 in 2010), but the number of suicides in the National Guard and the Army Reserve increased by 55 percent (80 in 2009; 145 in 2010).
- Mental illnesses and substance use disorders caused more hospitalizations among U.S. troops in 2009 than any other cause.[1]

According to the Departments of Housing and Urban Development (HUD) and Veterans Affairs (VA), nearly 76,000 veterans were homeless on any given night in 2009. Approximately, 136,000 veterans spent at least one night in a shelter during that year.[2]

Both from my perspectives as a patriotic American private citizen and as a chief of police who must manage a law enforcement agency to deal with the problems referenced by SAMHSA and HUD, I see these problems confronting our veterans as absolutely unacceptable in this day and age. It's easy to point a finger of blame at the DVA, whose offices are overwhelmed with veterans filing claims, but the larger problem is that communities themselves, and the law enforcement agencies that protect them, must step up to face the problem and help themselves by helping our veterans. For the police, we need

1 From the Substance Abuse and Mental Health Services Administration at http://www.samhsa.gov/veterans-military-families
2 VA & HUD Issue First-Ever Report on Homeless Veterans (2/10/2011) at http://www.va.gov/opa/pressrel/pressrelease.cfm?id=2053

special training in veterans issues and issues of mental health. For the courts, we need more comprehensive and better thought intervention programs. But we need better community mental health programs.

Mike Masterson, Chief of Police (Ret.),
Boise, Idaho, Police Department

Foreword by Peter Grimm

"Without force health protection, we cannot have force protection. . . . And without force protection, we can neither defend this nation in foreign wars nor defend its private citizens inside our own borders."

Wounded Minds examines the history and practice of recognizing and treating Post-Traumatic Stress Disorder ("PTSD"). It illustrates with potential examples the danger to individuals and society of failing to properly diagnose and treat PTSD and proposes solutions. *Wounded Minds* contains valuable insight for practicing psychiatrists, officials in Congress or the Veterans Administration, and even the general public. The current epidemic of "mass murders" in America makes this a timely topic, if only because most killings classified as "mass murders" are actually murder-suicides.

The stresses which can produce PTSD are not unique to our military. Those from abusive homes, those who have experienced bullying, those in the law enforcement community, victims of sexual abuse, and those who simply experienced an horrific event may all exhibit symptoms of PTSD. But those who have been to war are far more likely to acquire PTSD to a degree that is debilitating. One has only to realize that suicide rates among our military veteran population are nearly triple the national norm to understand this. And worse, those committing suicide often take others with them.

Dr. John Liebert has practiced clinical psychiatry for over fifty years. He began in the 1960s in the military and continues to this day in private practice. He has treated thousands of military and law enforcement personnel, many with symptoms of PTSD. The breadth and scope of his practice makes him uniquely qualified to report and critique the history of government policies with regard to PTSD, from initial denial to the current acknowledgement. It also makes his counsel extremely valuable in assessing the current state of evaluation and treatment and the way forward.

Peter Grimm is a West Point Graduate and field commander in Vietnam, awarded the Purple Heart. His family and personal roots run both deep and broad within The Long Gray Line of West Point grads.

Preface by Meg Kissinger

Wade Michael Page's Army buddies knew for years that he was a dangerously troubled man.

They feared he might kill himself. Yet, when they broke into his apartment one night and found him passed out drunk on the floor, they agreed to keep it quiet. That's what Army buddies do: they close ranks, protect one another.

"I wish now that we would have reported it," said Christopher Robillard, Wade's fellow psychological operations corp members.

Maybe if they had, Page would have gotten the help he needed. Maybe he would not have burst into a Sikh temple in Oak Creek, Wis., and killed six worshippers before turning the gun on himself.

As I groped to try and understand Page's motivations for the readers of the *Milwaukee Journal Sentinel*, I knew immediately whom to call. John Liebert is the nation's expert on the psychological trauma our military faces. A Vietnam veteran and psychiatrist, John screens military officers for their fitness to serve. His insight and advice have been critical in my efforts to make sense of these senseless acts.

The problems have only intensified since Page's rampage in 2012. There is more than one mass killing in America a day, many committed by veterans who suffered trauma while in service. Suicides by veterans began to spike to all-time highs in 2005 and continue their upward trajectory.

It's now a full-blown public health epidemic.

Liebert and his co-author William Birnes provide a desperately needed course on understanding the trauma our nation's troops suffer with the eccentricities and uncertainties that distinguish modern warfare. They walk us through the science of post-traumatic stress and describe in chilling detail the havoc that ensues when this is left untreated.

We need to come to grips with this crisis, and this book gives us a roadmap of how to do that. The casualties of modern combat mount long after these soldiers return home.

Like Page's buddies, we ignore these problems at our peril.

Meg Kissinger is an investigative reporter for the *Milwaukee Journal Sentinel* and the Eugene S. Pulliam Distinguished Visiting Professor of Journalism at DePauw University. She was a finalist for the Pulitzer Prize in investigative reporting and has won two George S. Polk Awards.

Chapter 1

What is Post-Traumatic Stress Disorder?

You may remember the character of James Bellamy from the PBS/ BBC television series "Upstairs, Downstairs." He returns from the front at the end of World War I as a changed man—after being shot at and gassed in the trenches, he has begun to suffer from a mental condition called "shell shock." That's what medical professionals called the mental state in which many soldiers found themselves after the war. They were still disoriented and socially dysfunctional because of their experiences during the war. Freud himself was perplexed by patients returning without physical disability from World War I and changed his entire construct for psychoanalysis from The Pleasure Principle to the instinctual conflict within all humans to live and procreate while self-destructing in returning to dust. Because of recurrent nightmares, he conceptualized the enigmatic compulsion to repeat the trauma—or repetition compulsion. For example, a woman raped at night in the park will feel compelled to revisit the park over and over again at night. This is certainly visible in victims of extreme psychological trauma and may be the seemingly futile effort to gain mastery over the unexpected and traumatic loss of control. Perhaps this is a fantasy, but perhaps, as with current practices of desensitization and implosion therapy for combat veterans, it can be natures way of healing from phobic avoidance of anything touching the senses from the original trauma, as in holding a weapon again.

In the motion picture *Patton*, General George S. Patton, Jr. (portrayed by George C. Scott), encounters a soldier in a military hospital in Italy. The man was trembling and crying that he couldn't take it anymore. Patton slapped him across the face, called him a coward, threatened to shoot him on the spot, and ordered that the soldier be taken out of a ward populated by other soldiers who had been wounded in battle. General Patton called him a coward, but the military doctors said he was suffering from a mental condition called "battle fatigue."

Now flash forward to the Vietnam War. This was a very different war from the two world wars of the first half of the twentieth century. Vietnam was also different from the Korean War—although the allies were ostensibly fighting the same ideological enemy (the Communist forces) the Korean War was a classic invasion from the north into the south; countries divided after the close of World War II. In Vietnam, however, the circumstances were very different, as the war was more of an insurgency than a classic invasion of one country by another. In fact, when the north invaded the south on June 25, 1950, it looked as though the outnumbered and outgunned South Koreans would be completely overrun, and the Communist forces would eliminate the sovereignty of the south. In response to the invasion, American forces stationed in occupied Japan were airlifted to a small section of territory in the southeast corner of the Korean peninsula, known as Pusan, and from there pushed their way north towards the 38th parallel (the dividing line between the two Koreas). It was a classic land invasion to gain a toehold for the purposes of establishing a perimeter from which to expand, just like the Allied landing at Anzio and later at Normandy. Vietnam was different.

In Vietnam—a war that President John F. Kennedy was trying to avoid by pulling out U.S. military personnel before he was assassinated—America and its allies were fighting an insurgent force backed by the North Vietnamese that had already defeated the French. In Vietnam, as many veterans of that war later told their doctors, you didn't know whom you were fighting until it was too late, because the very people you visited in villages said to be pacified by day turned into the enemy Viet Cong by night. It was challenging and frustrating, physically as well as psychologically, and for many, it caused mental derangement: Your friends, often guides known as "Kit Carsons," who had been former enemy combatants "re-educated" in South Vietnamese POW camps, sometimes turned on you, and the rules of engagement forced you not to shoot at those you knew, but couldn't prove, were the enemy. Yet, there were free fire zones where anything that moved could be killed—like killing fields that could later haunt our soldiers with guilt for killing innocents. It was a war that couldn't be won, a war that couldn't be Vietnamized, a war that lost its mission, and a war that destroyed the presidencies of John F. Kennedy, Lyndon Johnson, Richard Nixon, and Gerald Ford while compromising Jimmy Carter and Ronald Reagan until Bill Clinton decided to call the whole thing off and diapatched John Kerry to strike a deal with North Vietnam to grant them most favored nations status. Unless one called "Operation Phoenix," a clandestine operation that conducted kidnappings and assassinations of Viet Cong and North Vietnamese officials, a success, most American operations failed to blunt the North Vietnamese and Viet Cong war machine. American personnel listed as MIA or POW remained in Vietnam well after the war ostensibly ended in 1975 and probably still remain there today, just as American POWs remained in North Korea after that war and in the Soviet Union after World War I and II. They were soldiers left behind, according to James Sanders in *Soldiers of Misfortune*.[1]

---

[1] James Sanders, Mark Sauter, R. Cory Kirkwood, New York: Avon, 1994

In fact, the Vietnam War was so different from previous conflicts in the twentieth century that during the Tet Offensive in 1968 40,000 North Vietnamese troops and, reportedly, NVA General Giap himself, disguised as a refugee, infiltrated Saigon. The American military units were caught without weapons because no soldiers were allowed to carry weapons inside Saigon except for the 716th Military Police Battalion. The infiltration of Saigon was a near rout and disaster, according to some of the soldiers in Saigon who believed they were about to be overwhelmed. President Johnson said privately that the North Vietnamese success at Tet demonstrated to him that the war was unwinnable, and that in the face of a looming military disaster, he would not run for a second full term in office. We now know from the release of the LBJ Oval Office audio tapes that Johnson believed he was on the verge of negotiating an end to the US involvement in Vietnam. However, because, LBJ said, FBI Director J. Edgar Hoover told him that the Bureau had wiretapped the South Vietmanese ambassador to the United States, Hoover had learned that Republican presidential candidate and former vice president Richard Nixon had gone around the White House to convince the South Vietnamese not to go aong with LBJ and to hold out for a better deal with Nixon. In other words, the war could have ended in 1969 rather than in 1973. LBJ referred to Nixon's behavior as "treason" on the tapes. President Johnson who pushed the Civil Rights Act, Voting Rights Act, and Medicare through an adversarial Congress, was driven from office by the Viet Cong and the North Vietnamese. It was that kind of war—a war that ended with President Ford, Dick Cheney, and Donald Rumsfeld presiding over one of the most humiliating defeats and retreats of American military and diplomatic personnel in history, pulling frantic South Vietnamese clinging onto US Army helicopter landing skids for dear life, off the roof of the American embassy. When we think about who promulgated the war in Iraq, even before 9-11, it was Dick Cheney and Donald Rumsfeld, perhaps trying to restore what they lost as a result of the Vietnam debacle.

Like our war in Afghanistan—now a rear guard action in which our combat role is essentially at an end—Vietnam was a war in which the rules of engagement were very limiting, while the enemy wasn't at all limited. For example, patrols walked over spider holes connected to intricate and integrated fortified tunnels—deep underground tunnels, like the Tunnels of Chu Chi, that staved off the Japanese army. These tunnel complexes provided easy access to the Michelin rubber plantations, holdovers from the French colonial occupation and off-limits to U.S. troops, who were only allowed to engage in free-fire zones. Once the American patrols had walked past the spider holes, the Viet Cong (VC) had their backs. Then the VC would pop out of these spider holes and mow down our troops from behind. Michelin had agreements with our state department to avoid destroying their rubber trees while France had registered its opposition to the U.S. role in the war. Would it be surprising that VC found refuge there, just as the Taliban does in Pakistani tribal villages?

There were free-fire zones in Vietnam, where anything that moved could be shot. That was not always healthy, particularly if it was a farmer's water buffalo. There were also "no-fire zones," like the Michelin plantations. What kind of government would expose its youth to a war like this; a war in which you could be shot at, but often could not shoot back, even in self-defense? Booby traps on jungle trails were all but invisible, like roadside IEDs in the war on terror. The experienced point man—oftentimes Native Americans, by units' preference—might be good at detecting them. There is nothing naturally horizontal in the jungle. Tripwires were horizontal, and they were especially designed to spare the guy who tripped it and cause mass casualties around him. Wounded soldiers are a greater burden than dead soldiers because of the absolute necessity to treat the wounded. Americans took care of their wounded, and that made booby traps extremely effective. We have seen the same things in Iraq and Afghanistan—hence the high numbers of blast-related traumatic brain injuries and cases of Post-Traumatic Stress Disorder caused by our troops literally having to scrape dead bodies of their buddies off the exploded vehicles.

Vietnam was also a war that brought the problem of Post-Traumatic Stress Disorder (PTSD) to the forefront, because many returning veterans exhibited psychiatric symptoms that mystified many outside of the mental health profession. For example, why would veterans, even years after the war had ended, become nervous when they entered densely wooded areas? Why would some veterans exhibit severe antisocial tendencies, such as the recent Alabama murder, kidnapping, and hostage-taking by Vietnam War veteran and likely PTSD sufferer Jim Lee Dykes, who the military denies was ever in Vietnam? Why would some veterans be incapable of holding down jobs that required social interaction, describe suicidal ideations to family members or therapists, find themselves at odds with the criminal justice system, and wind up on the streets, homeless and begging for food? What had debilitated them to the point that many could no longer interact with the same society that had drafted them out of their homes, yanked them away from their families, and sent them marching off to war? The cause of the varying degrees of mental illness in many of those veterans was Post-Traumatic Stress Disorder, a condition that the military still agonizes over and struggles to diagnose correctly and then remedy.

Although it was bad forty years ago after the troops came home from Vietnam, it is far, far worse now as the troops return from Iraq and Afghanistan. In its own way, Afghanistan, a territory that has defied conquest for thousands of years, is much like Vietnam—so much so that the very people who lost the Vietnam War decided to relive it in Afghanistan, unfortunately with the same results. In addition, the epidemic of stress-generated suicides and homicides among returning veterans could well pose a greater threat to public safety than the terrorists our troops were sent to the Middle East to quell. Witness the very recent terror in the Southwest with ex-officer Christopher Dorner, who committed suicide in a cabin in the woods of Big Bear after murdering four people, and the execution-style double murders at the Glen Rose resort shooting range in Texas by Eddie Ray Routh, who had been diagnosed with PTSD.

In recent years, psychiatrists, psychologists, and allied mental health professionals have devoted an unprecedented degree of time and attention in an attempt to understand and treat people who engage in violent behavior. Previously regarded by many as untreatable, and hence suitable only for punishment from the criminal justice and penal systems or containment within psychiatric units, this population—and with it our understanding of the causes and prevention of violence—has begun to benefit from deeper neuroscientific understanding of the impact of trauma. They have also begun to heal as professionals recognize the shame, disorders of attachment, the complex grief over loss, the narcissistic injuries to self-esteem, and other issues that derive from the impact of trauma. Psychotherapeutic approaches that include empathy, object-relations, and the complex interactions between psyche, soma, and society have a profound impact on psychological functioning that is impaired by rage and murderous impulses resulting from psychic trauma, whether from war, childhood abuse, or oftentimes the volatile mix of both. The purpose of these approaches casts light on the causes, treatment, and prevention of violent behavior, not only in the context of forensic understanding and psychotherapy with violent individuals traumatized by war or in childhood, but also in psychotherapeutic relationships with those in the less traumatized population at risk for violence—i.e. the psychotic killer, such as University of Colorado Neuroscience grad student, James Holmes of the Aurora Theater Massacre, who had no history of psychological trauma.

There is substantial evidence that violence has its roots in trauma, and that it is a distinct form of aggression most often linked to the effects of childhood and adult trauma strongly determined and modified by complex variants in the person's genome. Trauma, although a given in battlefield situations, is far more widespread than has hitherto been acknowledged both in psychiatric patients and the general population. In other words, police officers, firefighters, children who grew up in abusive homes, spousal abuse victims, and survivors of near-accidents can all be subjected to trauma that results in post-traumatic stress. These findings are relevant to understanding why otherwise so-called "normal" people can become violent in certain situations under certain conditions.

To understand the root causes of how traumatic stress can instill violence against self as well as others, it is important to assess what is currently known about the traumatic origins of violence and how this can valuably inform the assessment process and treatment options—not only as they relate to the general population, but also for our warriors returning from combat.

Officially, Post-Traumatic Stress Disorder is a disorder of the human mind that has only been diagnosed and seriously researched in the past thirty years—five years after the evacuation of Saigon.In the Seattle Veterans Administration Medical Center in 1968, the wards were full of young veterans, but few, if any, psychiatry residents or staff psychiatrists ever mentioned combat trauma as a causative factor for these young veterans' admission to the hospital. Nor was it either necessary or a part of training to take combat histories from these young veterans or from the older veterans on the wards, many of whom were World War II and Korean War vets. The maverick chief resident, also coming right out of military service, said that he took combat histories from patients. He is the only one of scores of psychiatric and psychology trainees who did. Many psychiatrists from that period in the late 1960s felt embittered with shared guilt about the blindness imposed upon them at one of the top medical training institutions in the nation, the University of Washington. Many of these psychiatrists and residents in other specialties were products of the Vietnam doctor draft that also, ironically, occurred right after the assassination of JFK. It was known then that President Johnson was afraid of global turmoil, and particularly of a possible upheaval among Peace Corps volunteers worldwide. Their admiration and love for President Kennedy promised very unpredictable responses around the world from this cohort of young people. But Vietnam was still a very low-intensity theater of war when all doctors were drafted as interns nationally and dutifully boarded the buses for draft physicals in November 1963.

For these newly drafted interns—who would soon confront a psychological condition that would stymie the military for the next forty years—thirty-six hours on and twelve off was an inhumane schedule. Most interns were in their mid to late 20s, and some did not know what they were going to specialize in following their internships. When reporting for active duty on July 1, 1964, little had changed—except that fresh flowers marked the site of Kennedy's death on the route to San Antonio for military medical training, and active ballistic studies were still being done at the Texas School Book Depository. Vietnam was still an accompanied tour of duty where our servicemen could take their families. That would shortly change while they lined up for uniform allowances. For economically deprived interns, a roll of $300 in $50 bills was like a gift. For $100, they could buy an enlisted man's uniform, plan to borrow someone else's mess dress for formal occasions, and keep the $200 for luxuries not experienced in years, such as steaks at the Base Exchange grocery.

An occasional young doctor would step out of line and turn, reading his orders, "Where's Bien Hoa?" Another would ask, "Where's Tan Son Nhut?" The pronunciations, mixed with southern drawls and Brooklyn nasal twang, were memorable. Little did anyone in that line know what was awaiting them. Just days later, there was the Gulf of Tonkin incident, and all medical battle stations had been miraculously manned worldwide just in time for full scale war.

Colonel Franklin Jones was also busy drafting his policies and procedures for young men without college deferments who were about to be drafted and sent into guerilla warfare in the deadly jungles of Southeast Asia. "Anyone can take anything for one year" was the operational thinking back then. Colonel Jones spent the better half of his post-Vietnam military career touting the successes of reducing the evacuation rate of psychiatric casualties from over 20 percent in Korea to less than 1 percent in Vietnam. Immediacy and expectancy were the key words of Colonel Franklin Jones's psychiatric evacuation policy, and he would be taking its success with him to his grave. So these were the young men admitted to the Seattle Veterans Affairs Medical Center (VAMC), along with Veterans Affairs (VA) psych units nationwide. Jones's policies and procedures likely had an enduring impact on psychiatric directors of VA medical centers. Thus, "don't ask, don't tell" in the '60s and '70s applied to psychiatric practices in the VA, just as it did in the Army. There was no diagnosis for PTSD until the third edition of the Diagnostic and Statistical Manual (DSM) became the diagnostic driver for best practices.

A case in point: It was just after the Vietnam Tet Offensive, and Sergeant Wright was sent home from his assignment with the 527th MP unit on compassionate leave. His daughter had been hospitalized for an overdose. He presented in military uniform and was so pressured in his speech that his daughter's psychiatrist could hardly follow him. He was trying to convey the chaos of the Tet Offensive that had just occurred in Vietnam. The 527th MP was the only unit in Saigon allowed to carry weapons. Saigon was considered safe; every soldier had to check his weapon during leave days. But 40,000 North Vietnamese regulars disguised as refugees and simple visitors had infiltrated the city on foot and on bicycles. The fireworks of Tet broke out, but so did the gunfire.

It was a slaughter, because most of the U.S. troops, except for the 527th MP unit, were unarmed. In explaining this MP's experience of running through the streets in blood-soaked boots, a high-ranking staff member of the VA medical center rather sarcastically told the psychiatrist seeking help for this man, "Sounds like he has quite an imagination." The hubris back then was a disgrace, and worse yet, there was no diagnosis for this sergeant. Medic One came to the psychiatrist's office because the man collapsed on the floor with what appeared to be a heart attack. It was more likely a panic attack due to Post-Traumatic Stress Disorder. In the Diagnostic and Statistical Manual, published by the World Health Organization (WHO), there was a diagnosis for Sergeant Wright's problem, because Colonel Jones—all the names in this chapter are fictitious, by the way—had a lot of influence in the Pentagon, but not in the United Nations.

Sergeant Wright was diagnosed with Post-Traumatic syndrome under the then ICD diagnostic manual, and he never returned to Vietnam. He was medically discharged, but not with Post-Traumatic Stress Disorder, because back in the late '60s a diagnostic code did not exist for it in the Diagnostic and Statistical Manual, published by the World Health Organization (WHO). There was a diagnosis for Sergeant Wright's problem, because Colonel Jones had a lot of influence in the Pentagon, but not in the United Nations. PTSD was simply a mental illness that did not exist during the Vietnam War. It only exists today because veterans suffering from it have been presenting in numbers too large and too long for the bureaucracy to ignore. Now, bureaucrats have been accused of searching for pre-existing conditions so that the government won't have to financially compensate veterans for the rest of their lives since the advent of PTSD in the third edition of the American Psychiatric Association's Diagnostic Manual, DSM III.

In 1970, a Seattle VA psychologist had seemingly had enough of the deception and came to the psychiatric trainees, proposing a conference on "The Young Veteran." Of course, saying the word "Vietnam" back then would have cost him his position within the Department of Veterans Affairs. The conference was held, and a psychiatrist by the name of Dr. Mark Stuen—his real name—showed up from American Lake Veterans Hospital in Tacoma. Dr. Stuen had actually opened a unit at the hospital there to treat what he called "Post-Vietnam Syndrome." During his lecture, he described what we now know as Post-Traumatic Stress Disorder. Knowing that his program had a short life span with such a taboo diagnosis, he handed a stack of his unpublished manuscripts to a trusted colleague for safekeeping. They are probably now classics, although the manuscripts were never published. Dr. Stuen was right in his predictions for the future of his program.

When the diagnosis of Post-Traumatic Stress Disorder was finally officially recognized (although still marginalized) in the 1980s, the Department of Veterans Affairs developed PTSD programs within their hospitals, starting at Menlo Park VAMC in California. Later, Dr. Ray Scurfield started a program at American Lake VA hospital. It was sort of spooky, because Dr. Scurfield, standing on the ground of Dr. Stuen's Post-Vietnam Syndrome clinic, stated he had never heard of Dr. Stuen's program from the '60s. Post-Traumatic Stress Disorder is still highly politicized. The condition is often overdiagnosed to get high compensation for disabilities, and also underdiagnosed to save money for institutions like the military, VA, industrial insurers, and police departments, who avoid having to deal with its prevention—as may prove to be the case with crazed terrorist, former Naval officer, and ex-LAPD police officer Christopher Dormer, who committed suicide in a burning cabin in San Bernadino County, California after terrorizing the whole city on his rampage murders.

When a clinician sees a patient in emotional distress, there is a good chance that he or she has recently experienced an overwhelming psychologically traumatic experience, or is re-experiencing an older such trauma, perhaps years or decades past. No clinician can practice very long without seeing such a patient, because they number in the millions. For clinicians seeing men and women from a population of twenty million military veterans, the likelihood of seeing such a patient is 100 percent. The percentage of such clinical encounters in which a combat history is taken, however, falls dismally short of 100%, oftentimes matching the denial of the physician with that of the patient, who may present his distress in physical symptoms, rather than connecting emotional distress to long-ago comabat trauma and grief.

Most of these patients from the veteran population appear with a mood disorder, like panic attacks, anxiety, and depression. But what sets them apart from all other psychiatric patients and people in severe emotional distress are the following two symptoms: (1) Reliving the trauma and emotional overreactivity to external stimuli, like diving into the garden at a Fourth of July picnic when fire crackers go off; and (2) the actual, or automatic, drive of the human brain to shift them into emotional numbness and avoidant patterns of living to stop reliving and overreactivity, just like shifting a car into reverse to stop its forward motion from going over a cliff. The engine can jam up on the spot, just like the behavior of a PTSD sufferer.

It is this two-headed monster of life that is either too stimulus-bound by the irrelevant stimuli we all take for granted and ignore—such as a pile of dirt on the street, which in Iraq and Afghanistan could be hiding an Improvised Explosives Device (IED)—or the PTSD patients shut down emotionally by flooding their bodies with their own brain opiates and then avoiding normal life activities. Many Korean War veterans, for example, will find ways to surreptitiously isolate themselves until the snow melts; a snowy landscape is such an irrelevant stimulus triggering reliving of horrific winter battles. Of course, the severity, frequency, and duration of the trauma are matters of judgment for the clinician to determine, but we, as a human race, pretty much put the same relative values on stress and trauma. We are all bound by the similarities of our psyches, which, at a core brain-biological level, transcend cultural and racial differences.

Whether Japanese, Kenyan, British, or American, we humans rate death of a spouse far higher in numerical severity than losing a job.[2] And we know that the violent death of a loved one, whether by homicide or suicide, is extremely traumatic for anyone, regardless of culture, national origin, or country of residence. To diagnose Post-Traumatic Stress Disorder, there has to be a traumatic emotional experience outside the range of expectable life experience. We all

---

[2] Landmark study of Life Change Units on causation of disease and injuries by Holmes and Rahe, www.harvestenterprises-sra.com/The%20Holmes-Rahe%20Scale.htm.

lose our parents, and that is usually very stressful, even from natural causes late in their lives. But such loss, however stressful it is, is expectable. Finding a loved one hanging in the shower is not.

Judging trauma is essentially normal human experience that does not need a lot of education, but recognizing its impact on emotionally distressed patients does require clinical skills and training. Some patients who have been psychologically traumatized only become depressed or have severe anxiety, phobias, and panic attacks. But all of these emotional responses can cloak the essence of Post-Traumatic Stress Disorder and the reexperiencing of the trauma in numerous ways, such as in nightmares or actions that we frequently cannot remember either having or doing. Do victims of the Holocaust have nightmares? Probably, but often they cannot remember them. Do people turn off the road and forget why they are going somewhere? Oftentimes we do, and sometimes it's because we blacked out while passing something that reminds us of an emotionally traumatizing event, such as the spot where we know a loved one intentionally missed a curve, crashing into at tree at high speed. Then we come back to our awareness and discover that we are off course and should be driving to work. Such action is reliving of the traumatic experience, too, and this tends to transcend cultural diversity.

Just like the diagnosis of a visible or palpable event—such as a heart attack or stroke, where the symptoms are manifest, and the patient presents in predictable ways—we can make the same kinds of assessments with psychic injury caused by stress or psychological trauma, despite the differences in national and cultural definitions.

Post-Traumatic Stress Disorder and other stress disorders, unlike infectious diseases such as pneumonia or tuberculosis, are more arbitrarily defined by specific criteria in the patient's history, such as nightmares of the actual traumatic incident. There is no sample of bacteria of emotional trauma that we can test in a petrie dish, but we can interpret a patient's history and judge the severity of psychological trauma—an auto accident versus rape or sexual assault, for instance—trying to avoid excessive rigidity in eliciting and documenting necessary symptomatic criteria to meet the diagnosis. Such interrogative approaches can scare the patient into withholding his or her true emotional experiences. However, lacking standardized and validated objective testing for the pathological impact of stress and psychological trauma, controversy over diagnosis emerges when monetary considerations come into play as result of damages from war or second party liability, as in an auto accident. In other words, an insurance payer or the government will look to assess the validity of the patient's claims not because the patient's experience is in question, but because of payment guidelines and restrictions. A claims adjuster has to be responsive to his or her boss more than to the claimant. This is why so many veterans have a difficult time claiming PTSD from wartime experiences. Billions of dollars are at stake, and insurance institutions—as the Department of Veterans Affairs must in part be—view the claimant very differently than the attending physician. Often such disparate perspectives are driven by opposite motivations, such as screening out excessive demands for financial rewards in the former versus establishing a therapeutic alliance in the latter. Two doctors with similar credentials, therefore, might evaluate the same patient with different professional objectives. Too often their opinions collide, causing increased stress for the patient and costly administrative and adversarial medico-legal conflicts over financial compensation for the wound and its disability. They also are causing wait-times for initial claims review for nearly one million veterans of the war on terror approaching one year, even more than a year for New Yorkers.

However, psychiatrists who have to make the necessary diagnoses of PTSD rely on a set of objective criteria for that assessment. The criteria required for a clinician to make the diagnosis of Post-Traumatic Stress Disorder are as follows:

A. Exposure to a traumatic event
    1. Experience, witness, or be confronted with actual or threatened death or serious injury, or threat to the physical integrity of self or others
    2. Intense fear, helplessness, or horror

B. Persistent reexperiencing of the event
    1. Recurrent, intrusive, and distressing recollections of the event, including images, thoughts, or perceptions
    2. Recurrent distressing dreams of the event
    3. Acting or feeling as if the traumatic event were recurring (e.g., reliving the experience, illusions, hallucinations, and dissociative flashback episodes, including those on wakening or when intoxicated)
    4. Intense psychological distress upon exposure to internal or external cues that symbolize or resemble an aspect of the traumatic event
    5. Physiological reactivity upon exposure to internal or external cues that symbolize or resemble an aspect of the traumatic event

C. Avoidance of stimuli associated with this trauma and/or numbing of general emotional responsiveness
    1. Efforts to avoid thoughts, feelings, or conversations associated with the trauma
    2. Efforts to avoid activities, places, or people that arouse recollections of this trauma
    3. Inability to recall an important aspect of the trauma
    4. Markedly diminished interest or participation in significant activities
    5. Feeling of detachment or estrangement from others
    6. Restricted range of emotion (e.g., unable to have loving feelings)

7. Sense of a foreshortened future (e.g., does not expect to have a career, marriage, children, or a normal life span)

D. Persistent hyperarousal
   1. Difficulty falling or staying asleep
   2. Irritability or outbursts of anger
   3. Difficulty concentrating
   4. Hypervigilance
   5. Exaggerated startle response

E. The symptoms of criteria B, C, and D last for more than one month

F. The disturbance causes clinically significant distress or impairment in social, occupational, or other important areas of functioning

One must always remember the clinical judgment required to elicit and observe these criteria in a patient. And one must also know that a complex and tight construct for an abnormal clinical state is necessary for research, but it does not necessarily support effective diagnostics that inform best clinical interventions. We are talking about abnormal psychology that, by definition, likely manifests complex brain-based abnormalities, and we must—for now—rely on clinicians and evaluators to make criteria judgments based on their observations and histories from patients. These histories and observations, try as they might to be objective, are informed by the clinicians' experiences, both personal and educational, as well as pragmatically via their successes and failures in treatment. Therefore, they risk being subjective and catching the patient in adversarial medico-legal conflict, delayed compensation, and humiliation if the patient's recollections and claims are not believed. Obviously, few would disagree that we as clinicians need more objective diagnostic signs, such as brain-imaging abnormalities, to get beyond the subjectivity causing so many of the problems—espcially with claims processing of hundreds of thousands of combat veterans from the war on terror.

Within the abnormal human psychological states, known as psychopathology, specific discriminators must serve as tags for the meaningful mapping of clinical presentations. The descriptions of various symptoms and patient presentations create meaningful borders between the normal and abnormal. Presentations signaling either prototypical "mental disorganization" from flashbacks, or the classical triage prototype, "strange behavior" from emotional numbing, need to be separated from the dysphoria—emotional pain—of other conditions with "emotional distress." The DSM and its naming of specific descriptions of mental illnesses, therefore, provides clinicians with prototypes subject to more detailed refinement before qualifying them to either prescribe evidence-based treatment of PTSD or recommend a patient for financial reimbursement in long-term disability payments. Mentally disorganized and strangely behaving patients may neither solicit clinical help nor even have a chief complaint. In fact, statistics on completed suicides among combat veterans returning home demonstrate that the most lethal cases do not get clinical attention. Worse, clinicians report having seen soldiers with Post-Traumatic Stress Disorder who are as delusional as Schizophrenic patients, although they will not voluntarily come to a military clinic for assessment because of their delusions. They may live in isolation and merely be seen behaving strangely by others. The emotionally distressed patient, on the other hand, seeking relief from mental anguish, will do both. They both feel the pain and seek help.

Practicing psychiatrists are mainly occupied in Tertiary Prevention, which is the treatment of those already identified with severe enough impairment to reach the threshold of referral for psychiatric treatment. One might say, figuratively speaking, that Tertiary Prevention is pulling the bodies out of the river at the last bridge before they float out to sea and drown. Literally speaking, prevention of the most severe complications of psychiatric disorders requires preventing bodies from overwhelming our prison system—like Hasan and Bales—and their victims from going to the hospital and morgues, both here at home and in areas where we're fighting insurgency wars. Tertiary problems, except when the police bring in a violent offender, often drive a patient into a doctor's office, while underlying PTSD issues may fester for years just beneath the surface, only cropping up in times of stress. But, because PTSD can linger inside a person unless it's addressed in therapy and treated, the danger is that it generates emotional impairment severe enough that the impairment must be addressed by pulling back layers of issues before getting to the core problem. This is what some in our VA psychiatric program fear the most—namely, lifelong therapy and seventy-plus years of disability benefits in the millions, because of one incident in one battle. There are spokesmen for the government who state that this nation cannot afford the entitlements being claimed by hundreds of thousands of veterans. This leaves VA administrators with the quandary of what to do: Deny the claims of those who are mentally ill and send them into the streets or find ways to pay the entitlements regardless of budgetary constraints

Because of advances in brain imaging and in the understanding of the physiology of how post-traumatic stress works in the complex neurocircuitry of our brains, the possibilities that medication, combined with doctor/patient relationships, may become as well-grounded as treating a hernia when clinicians are able to resolve the stress issue biologically, as well as through psychotherapeutic interaction.

Chapter 2

Diagnosing and Understanding the Brain Abnormalities of PTSD

We view "mental states of unremitting human destructiveness"—whether to the self, to others, or both—from what is termed in modern psychiatric treatment as "brain-based" psychiatry. We start with modern knowledge of brain function and abnormalities to understand what might have driven these subjects to such catastrophic despair. Although still not advanced enough to diagnose the suicidal, violent, or post-traumatic patient—whether also head injured or not—modern neuroscience translated to brain-based psychiatry is too far along to simply "wing it" any longer with invalidated screening questionnaires and brief interviews that are obviously not working in the military. Nor have these questionnaires and cursory screenings ever worked in primary care, where studies show that

80 percent of completed suicides were preceded by a visit to the victim's primary care doctor, with documented notations indicating a desire to discuss suicidal ideation, plans, and intent. We need an approach that takes doctors into the biology of the brain and the neurological system. This is the newest frontier of brain science in neuropsychiatry, and it holds out enormous promise. Just in early 2013, it was reported that a team at NYU School of Medicine began a study to find what they are calling biological signals, called "biomarkers," that when analyzed, could provide objective evidence of invisible wounds, such as invisible war injuries.

Dr. Charles R. Marmar, chairman of the psychiatry department at NYU Langone Medical Center and lead investigator of the biomaker project, wants to find a mechanism that sets a standard for evaluating mental health in the same ways that doctors evaluate physical health. "You don't go from having shortness of breath to having cardiac surgery; you have a series of objective lab tests first," he said. "We would like to do the same thing with PTSD and TBI [traumatic brain injury]. That is, go beyond subjective reports."[3] Dr. Marmar's project is significant both because of its size—researchers hope to recruit 1,500 subjects,—but also because much of its financing is already guaranteed through a $17 million grant from the Steven A. and Alexandra M. Cohen Foundation.[4] Biomarkers are physiological road signs that can tell doctors whether a person has a disease or injury, or is likely to contract a particular ailment. Tissue damaged by a heart attack releases chemicals into the blood that can be detected. Abnormal levels of the proteins amyloid and tau, as well as the shrinkage of certain areas of the brain, are considered markers of Alzheimer's disease.

One intriguing brain-based finding in all well-diagnosed PTSD cases that have modern brain imaging performed is the shrinkage of an important brain structure deep in the interior of the brain;

---

[3] Shore, J. H., E. L. Tatum, and W. M. Vollmer. "Psychiatric Reactions to Disaster: The Mount St. Helens Experience." *American Journal of Psychiatry* 143, no. 5 (1986): 590-595.
[4] Reported in the *New York Times* by James Dao on February 6, 2013

the same structure necessary for normal memory and its loss in Alzheimer's disease. This is the hippocampus, and it shrinks in both well-diagnosed, recurrent major depression patients as well as in PTSD patients who are not clinically depressed. But, we are learning that trauma and its resulting effects on the brain are personalized. In a study of identical twins who both experienced combat stress, one soldier had PTSD, and the other did not. But, confounding the horse-and-cart question of brain abnormality findings in PTSD was the discovery that the unaffected twin had a normal-sized hippocampus. So, did the identical twin who did have well-diagnosed PTSD contract the disorder because of a small hippocampus? Or was his hippocampus shrunk by the repeated psychic hits of combat trauma? We cannot say definitively as of yet whether the small hippocampus is a congenital—or inborn—risk factor for developing PTSD in combat, or if it is a biological marker of the effects of repeated combat trauma on the brain. And, most importantly, this single twin study does not clearly match the traumatic combat experiences of these identical twin combatants. The soldier with PTSD and shrunken hippocampus may have been exposed to more horrific combat experiences, or of a higher intensity, or over a longer duration. We now know that the longer a soldier is exposed to traumatic events in combat, and the more intense those events are, the greater the likelihood that the soldier will be at risk for PTSD. But in the case of the twins, perhaps they are matched for genes, but not for environmental hits in the old "two-hit theory" of mental illness due to environmental trauma and genetic vulnerability. We know, for example, from studies of survivors of the Mount St. Helens's volcanic eruption, that Post-Traumatic Stress Disorder is dose–related. Dose-related means that the closer to the lava flow, the more the destruction of residences and the higher the incidence of PTSD.[5]

---

[5] Shore, University of Oregon study of survivors of Shore, J. H., E. L. Tatum, and W. M. Vollmer. "Psychiatric Reactions to Disaster: The Mount St. Helens Experience." American Journal of Psychiatry 143, no. 5 (1986): 590-595.

Translated into our discussion of PTSD in soldiers, the closer to a traumatic event and the greater the intensity of that event, the higher the incidence of PTSD. And, likely genes are both protective and weakening to human resilience in adapting to trauma because some genes predispose us to a weakened resilience to trauma while others may actually protect us at the time by providing a neurochemical numbing effect. This is more likely true to a point of no return, after which the trauma—such as that endured by Holocaust survivors— becomes primarily environmental, without much protection from any human DNA. Dr. Marmor's research promises many new avenues of discovery. Marmor's work is promising in that it allows measurement, and therefore determination of the severity of all known and suspected parameters of Post-Traumatic Stress Disorder.

It doesn't take an advanced professional degree to understand that stress and trauma go with life. In fact, the occurrence of traumatic events in human life in this country is remarkably high. Most people have experienced extreme trauma qualifying for one criterion of the disorder of Post-Traumatic Stress Disorder, which is an extreme, stressful event outside the range of expectable life experience. Becoming a crime victim is one such example. To that point, the lifetime prevalence of rape in women approaches 12 percent, but there is an enormous variability in the long-term disability from symptoms. The variability is likely due to more than the severity of the attack or genetic vulnerability; the professionalism of criminal justice and medical personnel in response to the attack is critically important. We have seen rape victims retraumatized by police and doctors who convey a sense of blame to the victim for being provocatively dressed, drinking before the attack, or dating the perpetrator, as in date rape.

Our primal stress and resiliency neurocircuitry and resulting reactions have not changed much since the first humans began populating the planet. The early Homo sapiens and neanderthal characters inhabiting Jane Auel's Caveman series have much the same physiological stress reactions to traumatic experiences that modern humans do. We don't live in caves, hunt bears, or flee from saber-tooth tigers on a daily basis, but our stress response has probably not changed that much, because today's saber-tooth tiger on the prowl for prey is perhaps now the mugger on the prowl for victims. The violent patriarchal chief of the cave clan unfortunately still exists in our society, despite its moves towards the equality of rights between the sexes; violent parents, boyfriends, or spouses still inflict traumatic damage on their victims.

From a biological and evolutionary perspective, we have the same stress response circuits in our brain and bodies as the real cave dwellers did even before the use of tools developed with the evolution of brain structure and human language. This primordial survival circuit starts in another brain structure deep in our brains very close to our hippocampus. We call this small, deep, and primeval region of the brain the limbic system. Harvard researcher Dr. Murray even called violence "limbic music" to trap the essence of flawed and maladaptive brain circuits tuned to live in caves, rather than go out on neighborhood watches. Florida murder suspect George Zimmerman claims to have stood his ground, but both sides are examining his limbic music for evidence of primary aggression or defensive aggression when killing Trayvon Martin.

Every day we can expect our stress response circuitry deep inside our primeval brain—the limbic system—to measure threat according to our hard drive memories of what is threatening or not. Dogs that have another tiny structure of their limbic system disabled, called the amygdala, actually yawn when a snake crawls over their paws. The human amygdala is programmed by primordial instinct, learning, and experience to recognize threat, and we are all different in this regard, although some threats, like being trapped by fire, are primordial. For example, the advancing wall of fire was a threat to everyone who saw it during the eruption of Mount St. Helens. The hail of fire from James Holmes's AR-15 assault rifle sent theater inhabitants in Aurora diving for the floor and fleeing for the exits as they tried to escape imminent death. But all who survived, the wounded and those who fled, will likely have some lasting post-traumatic stress reactions from the event, because it was a primordial threat. So what is the physiological system in our neurocircuitry that conveys this message, preparing us for fight or flight?

In the majority of otherwise nontraumatized human beings, a fight-or-flight primal threat response is governed by a small structure of our brain that is part neuron and part hormonal gland. It is the posterior pituitary portion of the brain's hypothalamus that spurts the cortisol releasing factor (CRF) hormone into a stalk connected to the anterior pituitary. This posterior pituitary brain structure is uniquely formed from both neuronal brain tissue and hormonal glandular. The anterior pituitary is endocrine hormonal tissue regulating adrenal, ovarian, testicular, and thyroid glands. Together they are known as the conductor of the endocrine, the hormonal orchestra of our bodies. And, for healthy stress response, these two lobes of the pituitary (hypophysis)—part brain and part endocrine hormonal tissue—are the default for our fight-or-flight mechanism, as common to the cave man as it is to us. Without its normal function in response to our perceived threat of stress, we are incapable of coping with life, particularly expectable stresses (such as last-minute Christmas shopping) and the unexpectable (such as surprise threats to our existence in the form of being attacked or mugged in the dark).

The cortisol releasing factor (CRF) from brain cells of the posterior pituitary stimulates the anterior pituitary to secrete adrenocorticotropic hormone (ACTH). This hormone is secreted in response to physical or emotional stress, especially low blood sugar; intense heat or cold; trauma, whether physical or psychological; surgery; immobility; and plasma cortisol levels. This release of ACTH is regulated through an intricate automated feedback mechanism that tells the pituitary, "There is too much, so shut down," or "There is not enough, so pump more ACTH." It bypasses intentionality and rational dominant-hemisphere control by something analogous to flying under our thought-processing radar. It responds to surprise threat before we have time to think about the nature of the threat, like the stick poked into one's back is a playful joke or life-threatening murder weapon. Regardless of what it is, the pituitary stimulates the adrenal glands to secrete cortisol, which stimulates the body cells, promoting protein breakdown, emergency glucose metabolism— which is why diabetics are urged to engage in rigorous exercise— and enhancing fat deposits for strengthened response to stress. This brain-hormonal circuit is and has been critically necessary for survival of humankind throughout the millennia. However, like any physiological system, it breaks down.

Normally, throughout the day, this mechanism automatically cycles from an embedded clock known as circadian rhythm, also controlled in part by brain-secreting hormones, like melatonin, as well as light. But it also changes with exposure to stress. When confronted with a threat, like a mugger jumping out of the doorway on a dark street, the hypothalamus orchestrates the release of more cortisol to gear us up for fight or flight. Our blood sugar levels go up to provide energy, our hearts pound faster to provide more oxygen, and our metabolisms shift from building protein to supplying us with the carbohydrates for energy. Assuming we survive the mugging and maybe only lose our wallet, a normal human stress circuit will quiet down and return to normal.

But what if our genes have created an abnormal "biased circuit" that activates the hypothalamus to pour out too much CRF, either in response to the threat, or after it is over and should start quieting down. Then, too much cortisone hits our hippocampus and the adrenal gland's hormonal message receptors. The hippocampus likely shrinks from the pounding caused by releasing too much cortisol, and the adrenal gland mistakenly responds by believing, through a regulatory feedback loop, that there is more than enough cortisol in the system. Thus, it shuts down. With the adrenal system in shut-down mode, the hypothalamus keeps pumping CRF, the hippocampus keeps shrinking, and we can't get the cortisol we need to confront the next stress. We are now in a diseased state: intolerant of stress, or perhaps totally avoidant of stress to the point of being homebound, agoraphobic or afraid—like many combat veterans— to leave home for shopping (hence, fear of the market). Markets are dangerous for soldiers in Iraq and Afghnistan because they have a lot of people, only one of whom needs to dial a cell phone to ignite a deadly improvised explosive device. It's no surprise, therefore, that some returning vets with PTSD have a fear of entering markets or even large department stores.

One can thus see how physiology and often-repressed memories— likely stored in the hippocampus—work together to produce a dysfunctional emotional reaction that's also physiologically based. Remember that the hippocampus is considered the critically impaired brain structure for memory loss in Alzheimer's disease. Without this section of the brain, there likely would not be PTSD, because people would not remember trauma. Moreover, brain structures communicate with each other through neurochemical and electrical signaling via neurocircuitry connections. Therefore, stimulating the emotional control neurons in the lower inside region of the frontal lobe—the ventromedial prefrontal cortex (VMPFC)— and the hypothalamus with the neurotransmitter, noradrenaline, from a cluster of neurons deep in the primitive human brain in turn stimulates that threat-awareness structure, the amygdala, to alert for threat. The amygdala has memory and can be tuned to the environment, as seen in the dog that depends on it to respond the right way to a snake crawling across its paws. The amygdala's primary function is to make animals aware of novelty, such as an unusual pile of dirt on the highway hiding an improvised explosive device, or a horizontal branch across a jungle trail that was a trip wire for a booby trap in Vietnam.

Thus is the combat veteran's amygdala similarly attuned. Firecrackers at the Fourth of July picnic are immediately processed as gunshots, and he/she dives—with later embarrassment—into the garden while relatives and friends are dumbfounded. "What's the matter with that guy?" What's wrong is that, because his amygdala was tuned for the right sounds in Mosul, Iraq, it cannot filter firecrackers from gunshots. Remember the 1968 Tet Offensive? Everyone was expecting firecrackers to open Tet, but the North Vietnamese infiltrators opened up with automatic gunfire. It didn't help our soldiers during Tet to know the difference between fireworks and gunfire. But, by blocking the stress response circuitry with what's called a beta blocker—like the medication, Inderal—the neurotransmitter, noradrenaline, cannot stimulate the hypothalamus and prefrontal cortex into pushing the amygdala's combat-tuned amygdala. Now, the returned soldier can sometimes maintain his sense of the present, knowing he is with friends and relatives at a party and is safe. He's back home and no longer in the combat zone. But it is the soldier who has trouble holding onto his sense of the present who is our immediate concern.

For example, when Eddie Ray Routh, now in custody, killed famous sniper and author Chris Kyle and his buddy at the range, forensic psychiatrists needed to determine whether his state of consciousness was in the present, or whether he had lost his sense of the present and was in combat mode, or in fact actual combat. The warrior within all combat veterans is a state of mind that probably never erases from the brain's hard drive. Parachute into Kandahar with that neatly tailored attorney walking with you to court, and you will suddenly see a different man: a warrior, immediately in combat mode for survival. The mental state doesn't go away. What happens when the warrior mental state is falsely called to action in civilian life are conditions that either make no apparent sense— such as diving into the bushes at a family picnic—or, in the case of Routh, are actually criminal acts, such as wrongly identifying and shooting someone in perceived self-defense. We are talking about someone we identify as the internal soldier, whose "animas," in Jungian psychology, becomes threatened by his own memories of combat. Within this soldier's neurological infrastructure, brain regions of the primitive brain try talking to each other to filter environmental messages as threat or safe, but sometimes they can't. That is the problem facing those institutions charged with protecting

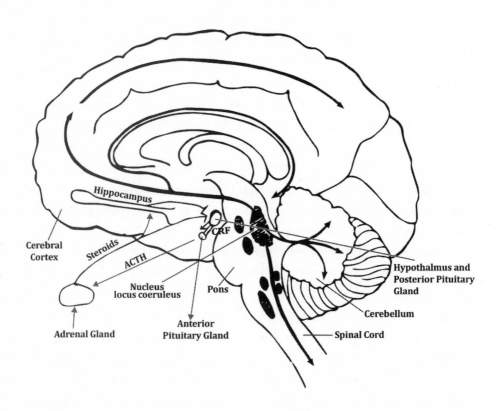

Normal circuitry, biased circuitry, and diabolical learning of neurocircuits responsible for "stress diathesis" showing the hypothalamus secreting GRF, which stimulates the anterior pituitary to secrete ACTH. This then circulates in the general blood stream to stimulate cortisol. Cortisol, in turn, informs the amygdala, and via feedback loop, the adrenal gland about what to do. This can either be normal response to stress or trauma, or it can be stress diathesis with shrinking of the hippocampus.

that soldier from himself, and in cases of extreme dangerousness, protecting society from that injured soldier.

Unfortunately for our soldiers and victims of extreme trauma, even normal circuits can become overwhelmed and work the same way, as we've seen with reactions from survivors of Japanese and German death camps in WWII. For these victims, no genetic empowering was strong enough to protect mind and body from PTSD. And, in Norwegian death camps, SS guards used blunt force to the heads of prisoners more than in other concentration camps, causing both concussive and subconcussive traumatic brain injuries.[6] Our soldiers, too, are coming home with physical traumatic brain injuries (both concussive and subconcussive), PTSD, or in many cases, both. We are also learning from medical research and the discovery process of lawsuits filed against the NFL that even well-trained athletes who suffer degrees of subconcussive brain injuries can have lasting traumatic effects that are eventually visible in premature deterioration of brain structure on imaging studies.

There is also the second injury in Post-Traumatic Stress Disorder, wherein the first injury is the actual combat trauma, and the second hit is the arbitrary and capricious disciplinary action requiring the soldier to prove he was actually in the battle he said he was. For example, in studying the history of Holocaust victims reporting their experiences in concentration camps, the first psychological injury came from the Nazis themselves. The second injury came from West German psychiatrists, who attributed their disability for compensation purposes to obsessive-compulsive disorder (OCD). In other words, in a larger context, it wasn't the Nazi arrests that resulted in emotional trauma, but a preexisting condition that many people have and function with on a daily basis, such as checking their locks compulsively three times every night. We see this today

---

[6] Ettinger on Norwegian Holocaust victims

in the way that military forensic psychiatrists attribute veterans' disability claims to preexisting condition so as to dismiss them.

There are allegations that military and VA psychiatrists diagnose personality disorders in order to disqualify returning combat veterans for their entitlements if disabled. There are many similarities between Borderline Personality Disorder and PTSD, especially in the tendency for breaking up relationships and impulsivity. And oftentimes, patients do have both conditions. But Borderline Personality Disorder is an enduring lifetime constellation of personality traits that would be obvious in boot camp and a likely disqaulifier for military service. Soliders with personality disorders certainly can make it into the military and survive combat; they can also acquire PTSD and blast injuries to the brain. But, Borderline Personality Disorder is not caused by combat. Traumatic brain injuries and Post-Traumatic Stress Disorder, however, are. Such diagnostic confusion, whether intentional or not, has no place in either military or VA psychiatry, and must end. Diagnostics must be valid, thus meeting the criteria of stability over time and predicting response to treatment and life events.

Individuals with Borderline Personality Disorder, for example, do not swerve off the highway when seeing a pile of rubbish on the curb, but combat veterans with PTSD do, and at great risk to their lives and the lives of others. Therefore, psychiatrists had better get it right or find a new occupation. With this critically traumatized population of young adults, diagnostic errors simply must be minimized. All causes of maladaptive behavior, such as blast injuries to the head and Post-Traumatic Stress Disorder, must be systematically ruled out before jumping to the conclusion that the veteran has always been character disordered and that four combat deployments did not alter that fact. For the combat veteran, like the incest victim, this is disavowal, as if to argue that it really didn't happen to you. Second injury is damaging. Psychiatry, whether military or VA, is supposed to help and not hurt, which necessitates extra caution in diagnosing combat veterans with preexisting personality disorders to avoid the risk of second injury by disavowing the tortured memory of the first injury.

In the two-hit theory we are discussing, we study environmental factors that precipitate traumatic events with an eye to examining how different types of people react to them. For example, there are differences between the sexes in both the frequency of encountering traumas and the likelihood of developing PTSD from them. In general, it is the less common—even rare traumatic events—that are most likely to predict ultimate onset of PTSD. For example, in women, a natural disaster, such as the massive tornado strikes in Oklahoma in 2012 that destroyed homes and towns, has a frequency of more than 12 percent every year, but the chances of the event being pathogenic and causing PTSD is 7 percent or less. Yet childhood physical abuse of females supposedly occurs with a frequency of 7 percent of girls every year, but predicts development of PTSD at 12 percent or higher in these victims. Similarly, with statistics among personnel in the military, 7 percent of men go to combat every year, but many more than 12 percent of them acquire PTSD from their military service.

These statistics tell the story of a VA and military health and disability insurance system that is overwhelmed and desperate for solutions. At the minimum, we can see that this calculation works out to over 250,000 veterans of our global War on Terror having reliably diagnosed PTSD. In fact, the number is likely higher, but even this minimal threshold figure loudly calls for attention from the highest levels of government, and the electorate, too. Few families today do not have a loved one or friend experiencing the problems of readjusting from combat in Iraq, Africa, or Afghanistan. And no family is totally isolated from a friend or loved one who is a combat veteran.

There are now 20 million veterans of foreign wars in this country, the vast majority of whom were in combat. Knowing this, we ask, how are our veterans and returnees from Asia and Africa going to be cared for? It is politically expedient, yet irresponsible, to believe any politician's promise to gear up VA and military medical services to take care of them. We know they are more likely to end up deteriorating, both physically and mentally—in isolation, getting thrown into prison, living on the streets, and committing suicide—than receive anywhere near the level of care they need to recover from the traumas of combat. The resources simply are not there. Preparedeness for the casualties of this war was not there. And it is too late to catch up with the damages. There simply are not enough resources to bring to bear on this public health crisis of our three million returning veterans—most of whom had multiple deployments—and few of whom, compared to previous wars, were in secure base settings. In the War on Terror, every day is Tet 1968. The only surprise is not being surprised by a sneak attack from the outside, or increasingly the inside, as ally Afghans turn on their NATO comrades-in-arms.

Knowing the statistics of at-risk soldiers suffering from the trauma of combat and the resulting disorder, can we pick out in advance those in that 12 percent and higher risk category for getting PTSD? To a certain degree we can—if they are child abuse victims, have a family history of psychiatric illness, or were likely to have a psychiatric illness. We have learned that, regardless of combat-induced trauma—or as has been too often the case with the volunteer army, psychiatric illness—before being recruited and enlisting, soldiers with prior issues of traumatic stress and resulting disorder or psychiatric illness are at high risk of developing PTSD in combat. Such risk factors include severe childhood family dysfunction as we often see in adult children of alcoholics. Stresses inherent in returning home include the realization that getting a job may be impossible, or the lack of social support from a combat unit that shared understanding and grief, or new traumas, such as drive-by shootings from gang-related crime. Studies of preexisting life experiences are either protective for soldiers in combat or significant risk factors for getting PTSD. Little, however, is known about female soldiers, whose exposure to combat in the War on Terror is unique in the U.S. military.

Physiological risk factors include a shrunken hippocampal brain structure and genetic abnormalities, causing biased neurocircuits incapable of processing trauma and stress, or processing different types of trauma differently. The latter, for example, brings up the issue of witnessing versus actual exposure to the trauma. Soldiers who witnessed atrocities, but did not participate in them, are more often numbed and in denial, rather than actively reliving the atrocities with flashbacks and nightmares—although witnessing the atrocities will also produce PTSD in a percentage of witnesses.

There is a threshold for what anyone can take. It was once believed by the Defense Department that anyone should be able to take anything for one year. We soon learned that Vietnam battle experience was a glaring exception, resulting in an overwhelming epidemic of PTSD. That epidemic lingers today among Vietnam vets still struggling to find peace with themselves, vets who never even received public recognition for their service until over a decade after the war ended.[7]

We know that early childhood stress and child abuse is an environmental hit that predisposes the adult to risk of getting PTSD from later trauma, such as combat.[8] The most likely cause of this increased vulnerability to adult PTSD from bad childhood experiences—whether the stress of dysfunctional family life, as in multiple divorces of parents, or the trauma of sexual or physical abuse—is the deregulation of the normal stress-response neurocircuitry, whether a burned-out circuit insensitive to stress or an over-activated circuit needing just one more hit, as in combat, to

---

[7] World Congress of Psychiatry, Military Section, Franklyn Jones, MD, US Army on reduced expectations of evacuation from combat zone in VN and John Liebert, MD, "Psychogenesis of Brutality in Violent Occupations".

[8] Liebert and Holiday, "Prevention of Stress Disorders in Police and Military Personnel", Proceedings of the FBI Academy Behavioral Science Unit Conference on Critical Incidents in Law Enforcement, 1989.

spin out of control. Of interest, however, is that many children who have similarly adverse events in early life are as resilient to trauma as adults as those growing up in relatively normal families. Therefore, one must question whether early childhood stress immunizes the person to later life trauma, or makes him/her more vulnerable. Much of this, of course, will depend on the type and severity of trauma and stress. Growing up as an older child in a family with multiple divorces, custodial parents, and foster placements might increase a person's resiliency to trauma, while being sexually abused by a father or close male relative makes the soldier more predisposed to PTSD from combat. Many adult children of alcoholics and victims of parental rage and sometimes physical abuse may outwardly appear resilient to stress but can have deeply embedded PTSD reactions if external stimuli push sensitive buttons. We have seen this in combat veterans as well. Research is needed, therefore, on the types of early childhood stresses that can have lasting effects on adults and on father-child incest. Incest is significantly under-reported in all populations and especially in the military population returning home from the war on terror.

This question of what types of trauma can lead to long-term PTSD also leads directly to what might be going on in our genes. There are likely genetic changes in childhood survivors of abuse that affect chemical messaging of cortisone within the brain and glandular stress response system. There are genetic abnormalities in the genes that regulate brain dopamine levels, causing too much or too little to be released in response to stress. Dopamine is a major neurochemical that mediates emotional response through brain function and is likely necessary for adapting to the excitability of war. Similarly, there are genetic abnormalities for brain serotonin, another neurochemical messaging system under stress. Most likely, this needs to be in balance with the excitatory effects of dopamine in order to cool off after combat. Normal serotonin and dopamine transmission within the brain is necessary for balanced brain function, and presumably maintenance of normal stress response in face of trauma. Finally, there is a brain protein, BDNF—brain-derived neurotrophic factor—which is known to activate and support repair and healthy alterations of neuronal pathway growth. BDNF is likely necessary for maintenance of normal stress response, and there can be genetic abnormalities that reduce the effectiveness of this neuronal protein. We still need to continue serious research into whether, and how, external abuse stimuli during early childhood can affect a young person's genetic makeup, so as to make him or her less resilient to stress as an adult. Here's why.

We still do not know, for example, whether all or only some of these changes are inborn or occur under environmental stress. We do know that recurrent depressive mood episodes in experimental animals leads to damaged DNA. It is possible, therefore, that early life trauma can damage genes. Yet, certainly, many people are simply born with one, some, or all of these genetic risk factors, preventing normal fight-or-flight stress response in the neurocircuitry handed down to us from our cavemen ancestors. Unfortunately, pre-recruitment screening and fitness for duty exams cannot pick up genetics prior to deployment, but this is a field for research to determine resilience to trauma.

How do all these risk factors assess the risk to the soldier for developing PTSD? In the War on Terror, we see unique stresses not previously encountered in other wars, and we have the trauma of combat—oftentimes more, less, or similar to that seen in any other war (The Faces of Battle, Keegan). But, with most soldiers now facing multiple tours—for some, four or more—there is the stress of the separation from loved ones, often ending with disastrous Dear John letters or returning home to a spouse's infidelity. Unique to the current war in Afghanistan, the super-high life-or-death tension of distinguishing an insurgent from an ally and the multiple successive or concurrent deployments simply allows no time or place to decompress from battle fatigue and hypervigilance. For example, your Afghan guard has to be assumed to be a Taliban in disguise, or an Afghan police officer may turn his weapon on you—as happens all too many times—thus requiring your buddy to stay awake while you sleep. Who's your ally? Who's your enemy? You can't tell them apart until it's too late. This is a unique stressor of war for our military.

Soldiers described the Vietnam War as "360," which meant there was no front line during patrols. But, if adequately defended with perimeter force protection, the forward operating base was safe inside from the enemy, if not from fraggings as revenge for a lieutenant taking excessive risks for career advancement and thus jeopardizing soldiers. Reportedly, many infantry lieutenants killed in action had an American bullet in their backs. But, assuming there was a good lieutenant under good command with the best of force protection for the perimeter, soldiers returning from patrol to their forward bases in Vietnam could stand down for a while, sleep, relax to some degree, decompress, let their pain and muscle strain subside, and let their stress response neurocircuitry settle down a bit to rejuvenate for the traumas and stresses of the next day's patrols. That is not the current state of affairs in Afghanistan, and it wasn't in Iraq, either. Remember the suicide bomber who blew up the mess hall in Mosul? He strapped a bomb to himself, dressed himself in an Iraqi uniform, walked into the mess hall on a U.S. base, and killed 14 American soldiers while wounding 89 others. For General Richard Meyers, the Chairman of the Joint Chiefs of Staff at the time, that was a game changer, as President Bush had already declared "mission accomplished."

The surprise element and gruesome horror of this attack in Mosul could have likely left no survivor without PTSD. This is the face of battle probably not even contemplated by Keegan in his graphic portrayal of destruction faced by soldiers in combat. These soldiers in Mosul were not in battle. They were eating in a supposedly well-defended forward operating base. One army psychiatrist never left the hospital in Mosul: His ability to empathize with those in combat is questionable, as he avoided combat exposure during his entire deployment, returning to pass judgment of soldiers' trauma and their responses to it with diagnostics for many that determined their fates throughout their lives.

Looking at the upward trend of PTSD risk factors in our Middle Eastern and Central Asian wars, both the unpredictability of events and Freud's own necessary element for post-traumatic syndromes— that of surprise—escalate in the final stages of the ground battle that is our global War on Terror. Our American rear guard is fighting a retreating battle to attain peace with honor in Afghanistan—an increasingly unlikely goal to achieve, as fewer troops are left under the protection of more Afghans whose loyalties are questionable at best. The specter of the retreat from Saigon also hangs over the retreat from Kabul. No president wants to watch a rout of his soldiers on CNN. NATO forces are responsible for what happens in Afghanistan, but Pakistan and Iran have more control over what happens, and even how we get out, because Afghanistan is landlocked by nations of questionable reliability in the event of our need to withdraw rapidly.

Unfortunately, like Vietnam and *Operation Iraqi Freedom*, the public support for these soldiers back home, and in the country of those they are trying to save from evil forces, is nil. They were sent off to war without adequate body protection armor, bullet-proof helmets, and protective armor for the vehicles that were exploding every day from roadside bombs. Remember the almost sardonic grin of then Defense Secretary Donald Rumsfeld as he gleefully explained to a seemingly lobotomized press corps that, "You fight a war with the army you have, not the army you don't have." Even Sun Tzu, author of the ancient Chinese Art of War, would have walked out of that press conference in disgust. It took us years to equip our troops adequately, even as we threw more of them into combat while private donors, such as the singer Cher, provided protective equipment for our troops.

Now that one of the Middle Eastern wars has ended de jure—and another war is set to end officially in 2014—the troops are coming home. However, the convenient political rhetoric on behalf of our heroes is not backed by real support from either the public or institutions funded to provide support to our returning troops. Upwards of a million vets are awaiting examinations at VA medical centers for injuries they believe to have suffered in combat. The wait is up to a year. Very recently, the public saw a veteran selling all his medals on eBay just to pay for groceries to feed his family. Just weeks ago, another veteran with PTSD, during an informal gun-range therapy session with two former Navy SEALS, shot and killed both former SEALS and fled in their pickup truck. Where was that veteran's support network? And more of his combat buddies are still in Afghanistan to fight the rear guard action, while many deactivated troops, separated from the military by choice or force, find themselves suffering alone, staring at guards from behind prison bars, begging on street corners for loose change, and sleeping in alleys, if they have not already taken their own lives.

One must ask whether politicians are exploiting these warriors for their own personal goals, while either doing nothing to help them, or worse yet, undermining institutions that could help by cutting their budgets at the very time need is highest. How easy it is to vote for a budgetary sequester when you're not the one being sequestered. Our civilian population and its leadership is completely divorced from a war they voted and paid for, yet know precious little about.

Never has there been a war started and led by so many civilian politicians who've never known—or are even reading about—the face of battle. It is showing in all the adverse consequences of lack of treatment, misdiagnosis, and even illegal alterations of PTSD patients' medical documents. Soldiers returning from combat have even been discharged from a psychiatric ward, escorted by MPs to the nearest homeless shelter, and simply dropped off there, no longer the Army's responsibility. That is disgusting to witness. But it is the harsh reality of a war led at the top by people with no experience in war for a population that largely has little or no experience in war, or individuals that are too traumatized themselves from Vietnam and Korea to be of help.

The soldiers' civilian peers simply believe that multi-tour combatants in the global War on Terror made the choice to volunteer, and therefore must put up with the consequences. The lack of support and dearth of resources for the returning troops, however, is shameful, which is why even the most liberal of news pundits are calling for the Pentagon to do something to show appreciation for veterans returning to the cold reality of an economy stuck in recession. And while these young men and women come home, they witness the government that sent them—and keeps sending them—to war held hostage for political gain by a coldly calculating Machiavellian Congress.

Families are not much better off when it comes to understanding the nature of the support returning veterans need, especially those suffering from undiagnosed PTSD. Particularly bad off are the employers of the institutions designed and funded to assist in veteran readjustment, because little or nothing is done by those initiating the ground actions of the War on Terror to assist returning soldiers in their readjustments in a meaningful way. In fact, the recent scandal of arbitrarily altering diagnoses at Madigan Hospital, which we deal with below, and the closure of the PTSD treatment unit there sends a strong signal to the soldier returning from our War on Terror. "You volunteered for this. You got paid. Now, it's up to you to find your own way—you can stay in the army or you can be discharged." And, as one psychiatrist at Madigan always told those he rejected for benefits, "Thanks for your service."

Focusing on what we know about the lack of veteran support and the brain-biology mechanism for Post-Traumatic Stress Disorder and other psychiatric illnesses, we have to look at the context of research into PTSD and what can be applied to the crisis of returning veterans in need of psychiatric help. With all the understanding we have acquired in the short time since Post-Traumatic Stress Disorder was even recognized as a brain-based clinical entity and disorder of the mind, clinicians need the bright lines of symptoms and signs to separate PTSD patients from others with similar emotional distress, such as mood and panic disordered patients. In medicine, this is called a differential diagnosis.

Chapter 3

Christopher Dorner in the Burning Cabin

Remember the 1994 OJ Simpson slow-speed car chase along the Los Angeles freeways, the fleet of LAPD and CHP black and whites with their lights flashing as they followed the accused, but now acquitted, killer of his wife Nicole and Ron Goldman winding his way through hills and canyons of Los Angeles County? Now flash forward to 2013 as similar images of tactical formations of police units from all across southern California tracked former LAPD and US Navy officer Christopher Dorner, perpetrator of a frightening killing spree, who made his way from the warm waters of San Diego to an isolated cabin at Big Bear Lake where he would make his final stand. What was behind his murders, the individuals he chose as targets, and his rage at the people and the institutions he claimed had wrecked his life? He tried to explain it all in the manifesto he posted online, a rant that revealed the depths of his insanity that was so meticulously laid out in its delusions of persecution, readers flocked to his support. Insanity can be that powerful. Dorner wrote:

Those who know me personally may find it hard to believe media reports stating I am suspected of committing such horrendous murders, and have taken drastic and shocking actions in the last couple of days. You may be saying to yourself, this is completely out of character for a man who always wore a smile wherever he went. I know I will be vilified by the LAPD and the media. Unfortunately, this is the necessary evil I must endure in order for substantial change to occur within the LAPD and to reclaim my good name. The department hasn't changed since the days of the Rampart scandal and Rodney King; it has gotten worse. The consent decree should never have been lifted. The only thing that has resulted from implementing the consent decree is that those officers involved in the Rampart scandal and Rodney King incidents have since been promoted to supervisor, commander, command staff, and executive positions.

The question is, what would you do to clear your name?

Name: A word or set of words by which a person, animal, place, or thing is known, addressed, or referred to.

Synonyms for "name": reputation, title, appellation, denomination, repute.

A person's name is more than just a noun, verb, or adjective. It's your life, your legacy, your journey, your sacrifices, and everything you've worked hard for every day of your life. You should never let anyone tarnish that name when you know you've lived up to your own set of ethics and personal ethos.

In August 2007, I reported an officer (Officer XXXX/now a Sergeant) for kicking a suspect (with excessive force) while I was assigned as a patrol officer at LAPD's Harbor Division. While cuffing the suspect (XXXX), XXXX kicked the suspect twice in the chest and once in the face. The kick to the face left a visible injury on the left cheek below the eye. Unfortunately, after reporting the incident to supervisors, and an investigation by PSB (internal affairs investigator Det. XXXX), nothing was done. I had broken their supposed "Blue Line". But it's not about JUST US on the force, it's about JUSTICE!!! In fact, 10 months later on June 25, 2008, after successfully completing probation, acquiring a basic Post Certificate, and Intermediate Post Certificate, I was relieved of duty by the LAPD while assigned to patrol at Southwest division. It was clear to me that the department was retaliating for my reporting of XXXX for kicking Mr. XXXX. The department stated that I had lied and fabricated the report of XXXX kicking the suspect.

I later went to a Board of Rights (BOR), a department hearing for a decision on continued employment, from October 2008 to January 2009. During this BOR hearing, a video was played for the BOR panel in which XXXX stated that he was indeed kicked by Officer XXXX (a video that was sent to multiple news agencies). In addition to XXXX stating he was kicked, his father, XXXX, also stated that his son, upon release from custody, had relayed that he was kicked by an officer during arrest. This was all presented to the department at the BOR hearing. Still, they found me guilty and I was terminated.

What wasn't mentioned was that the BOR panel, made up of Captain XXXX, Captain XXXX, and City Attorney XXXX, had a significant conflict of interest from the outset: Captain XXXX was a personal friend of XXXX from time as her supervisor at Harbor station. While this created a clear issue of objectivity, my argument for his removal from the BOR panel was denied. The advocate for the LAPD BOR was Sergeant XXXX. XXXX, however, also had a clear conflict of interest as she was XXXX's friend and former patrol partner at Harbor division. I made an argument for her removal when I discovered her relation to XXXX, and it was again denied.

During the BOR review, the department attempted to label me, unsuccessfully, as a bully. They stated that I had bullied a recruit, XXXX, in the academy, when in reality a deposition from the official 1.28 formal complaint investigation found that I had stood up for XXXX. (Other recruits had sung Nazi Hitler youth songs about burning Jewish ghettos in WWII Germany since XXXX's father was a concentration camp survivor.) It is appalling that they would attempt to label me with such a nasty, vile word. I would ask that journalists investigating this story ask Officer XXXX about the incident, since Officer XXXX was one of those singing along.

The internal affairs investigation into the academy involving XXXX was rejected based on a complaint that I had initiated hostility toward two fellow recruits/officers. While assigned a footbeat patrol in Hollywood Division, Officers XXXX and XXXX (both current LAPD officers) decided that they would voice their personal feelings about the black community.

While traveling back to the station in a twelve passenger van, I heard XXXX refer to another individual as a "nigger." I wasn't sure if I had heard correctly, since he was sitting in the very rear and I was in the front with at least eight other officers talking in between us. But, even with the multiple conversations and ambient noise, I again heard Officer XXXX call someone a nigger. Now that I had confirmed it, I told XXXX not to use that word again. I explained that it was a well-known, offensive word that shouldn't be used by anyone. He replied, "I'll say it when I want."

Officer XXXX, a friend of his, also asserted that he would say the word "nigger" when he wanted. At that point, I jumped over my front passenger seat, and two other officers, and placed my hands around XXXX's neck and squeezed. I stated to XXXX, "Don't fucking say that." At that point, there was pushing and shoving and we were separated by several other officers. What I should have done was put a bullet in his, and Officer XXXX's, skull. The situation would have been resolved, effective immediately.

The sad thing about this incident is that when Detective XXXX from internal affairs investigated, only one officer (unknown) in the van, other than myself, had a statement consistent with actual events. The other six officers all stated hearing and seeing nothing. Everyone involved should be ashamed, especially Detective XXXX (who is the same ethnicity as XXXX) for creating a separate 1.28 formal complaint against me (XXXX complaint) in retaliation for initiating the complaint against XXXX and XXXX. There shouldn't be retaliation against an honest officer for breaking the so-called "blue line." I hope your son XXXX, who I knew, is a better officer than you. Detective XXXX. The saddest part of this ordeal was that Officer XXXX and XXXX were only given 22 day suspensions and are still, to this day, LAPD officers.

Effectively, the LAPD stated that it was acceptable for officers to call fellow black officers "niggers" to their face, and all you'll receive is a slap on the wrist. Even sadder is that during the 22 day suspensions of XXXX and XXXX, the Los Angeles Police Protective League (LAPPL) paid the officers their salaries. When I received a two-day suspension for an accidental discharge, I took my suspension and never applied for a league salary. It's called integrity.

I would challenge journalists to investigate every residence I've ever had and find one instance where I was guilty of bullying. You won't because none exist. It's not in my DNA. Growing up, I was the only black kid in each of my classes, from first grade in elementary school to seventh grade in junior high, and any instances of being disciplined for fighting occurred in response to fellow students provoking schoolyard fights, or calling me a "nigger" and other derogatory terms. I grew up in neighborhoods where blacks constitute less than 1% of the population.

My earliest recollection of racism is from the first grade, while attending Norwalk Christian elementary school in Norwalk, Calif. A fellow student, XXXX if I recall, called me a nigger on the playground. My response was swift and non-lethal. I struck him fast and hard with a punch and a kick. He cried and reported it to a teacher, the teacher reported it to the principal, and the principal swatted XXXX for using the derogatory word. He then, for a reason unknown to me, swatted me for striking XXXX. He stated that as good Christians we are to turn the other cheek, as Jesus did.

The problem is, I'm not a fucking Christian and that old book called the Bible, which is fiction and limited nonfiction, never once stated Jesus was called a nigger. I thought, how dare you swat me for standing up for my rights, for demanding that I be treated as an equal human being. That day I made a life decision that I would not tolerate racial derogatory terms being spoken to me. Unfortunately, I was swatted multiple times for the same exact reason up until junior high. Terminating me for telling the truth concerning a Caucasian officer kicking a mentally ill man is disgusting.

Don't ever call me a fucking bully. I want all journalists to utilize every resource at their disposal that specializes in research collection for their reports. Through the discovery of available evidence, they will see the truth. Unfortunately, I will not be alive to see my name cleared. That's what this is about, my name. A man is nothing without his name. Below is a list of locations where I resided from childhood to adulthood.

Cerritos, Calif. Pico Rivera, Calif. La Palma, Calif. Thousand Oaks, Calif. Cedar City, Utah. Pensacola, Fla. Enid, Okla. Yorba Linda, Calif. Las Vegas, Nev.

During the BOR, an officer named Sergeant XXXX from Los Angeles Port Police testified on behalf of the LAPD. XXXX stated for the BOR that he arrived at the location of the UOF (Use of Force) shortly before I cuffed the suspect. He also stated that he assisted in cuffing the suspect and then told the BOR that he told me to fix my tie. All of those statements were LIES!!! XXXX, you arrived at the UOF location nearly 30 seconds after I had cuffed Mr.XXXX. All you did was help me lift the suspect to his feet, as it was difficult for me to do so alone because of his heavy weight. You did not tell me to fix my tie, as the BOR members and everyone else that was in the room know. It's clear you lied because the photographic evidence from the UOF scene, where XXXX's injuries were photographed, clearly shows me wearing a Class B uniform on that day.

A Class B uniform is a short sleeved uniform blouse. A short sleeved uniform blouse for the LAPD does not have a tie included. This is not a Super Troopers uniform, you jackass. Why did you feel the need to embellish and lie about your involvement in the UOF? Are you ashamed that you could not get hired on by any department other than port police? Do you have delusions of grandeur? What you did was perjury, which is exactly what XXXX did when stating she did not kick XXXX.

What they failed to mention in the Board of Rights (BOR) was XXXX's own use of force history during her career with the LAPD. She has admitted that she has a lengthy use of force record and has been flagged several times by risk management. She even has a very well-known nickname, Chupacabra, which she was very proud to flaunt around the division.

She found it very funny and entertaining to draw blood from suspects and arrestees. At one point she even intentionally ripped the flesh off the arm of a woman we had arrested for battery (she sprayed her neighbor with water from a garden hose). Knowing the woman had thin, elastic skin, XXXX performed an Indian burn on the woman's arm after cuffing her. That woman was in her mid-70s, a mother and grandmother, and was angry with her tenants who failed to pay rent on time—something I can completely understand (and I am sure many landlords have wanted to turn the hose on tenants who do not pay their rent).

XXXX was also demoted from a senior lead officer rank/position for performance issues. During my two months of working patrol with XXXX, I found her to be a very angry woman and learned that she had been pulled from patrol for a short time due to a domestic violence report made by the Long Beach Police Department involving an incident with her active LAPD officer boyfriend, XXXX.

XXXX is the same officer who has also been investigated for witness tampering. Additionally, she was visibly angry on a daily basis because she was going to have to file for bankruptcy (her ex-husband, a former LAPD officer and not XXXX, who had left the department, state, and was nowhere to be found, had left her with a tax bill and debt that she was unable to pay because of a lack of financial means). XXXX, you are a POS and you lied right to the BOR panel when XXXX asked you if you kicked XXXX. You destroyed my life and name because of your actions. Time is up. The time is now to confess to Chief Beck.

I ask that all journalists investigating this story submit requests for FOIA with the LAPD to gain access to the BOR transcripts, which occurred from October 2008 to February 2009. There, you will see that a video was played for the BOR members that showed Mr. XXXX, who suffers from Schizophrenia and Dementia, stating that he was kicked by a female officer.

That video evidence supports my claim that XXXX kicked the suspect twice in the upper body and once in the face. I would like all journalists to also request copies of all reports I wrote while employed by LAPD—whether in the academy, or during my 3 years as a police officer. There are DR#s attached to each report (investigative report) that I have ever written, so they all exist. A FOIA request will most likely be needed to access these at Parker center or at the Personnel/ Records.

You can judge my writing and grammar skills for yourself. The department attempted to paint me as an officer who could not write reports even though Sergeant XXXX, the training officer who trained me, stated for the BOR panel that there was nothing wrong with my report writing, and said that I was better than all rookie/ probationer officers he has ever trained. Officer XXXX stated the same, but refused to testify (as he did not want to "get involved" with the BOR's). Contact Sergeant XXXX, (now a Captain at Lompoc PD), Sergeant XXXX, and Sergeant XXXX. All will state that my report writing was impeccable.

I will note that I always typed my reports because I have messy handwriting/penmanship. However, I never had a single kickback/redlined report at Southwest division, and Sergeant XXXX and Sergeant XXXX can testify to that. I never received an UNSATISFACTORY on any day or week. The same can be said about my time with the U.S. Naval Reserves. All commanders will state that my report writing was always clear, concise, and impeccable. You can even search my AAR (after action reports), chits, memorandums, and IIR's (Intelligence Information Reports), which were written in the Navy. All were pristine.

I had worked patrol at LAPD's Harbor Division from February 2006 until July 2006, at which time I was involuntarily recalled back to active duty (US Navy) for a 12-month mobilization/deployment to Centcom in support of OIF/OEF. I returned to LAPD's Harbor division in July of 2007 and immediately returned to patrol. I worked at Harbor Division until November 2007 when I transferred to Southwest Division. I worked at Southwest Division until June 25, 2008 when I was relieved of duty.

I have exhausted all available means of recovering my name. I have tried all legal actions within the appeals process at the Superior Courts and California Appellate courts. This is my last resort. The LAPD has suppressed the truth, and it has led to deadly consequences. The LAPD's actions have cost me my law enforcement career, which began on Feb. 7, 2005 and ended on Jan. 2, 2009. They cost me my Naval career, which started in April 2002 and ended February 2013. I had a TS/SCI clearance (Top Secret Sensitive Compartmentalized Information) up until shortly after my termination with LAPD.

This is the highest clearance a service member can attain other than a Yankee White TS/SCI, which is only granted to those working with and around the President and Vice President of the United States. I lost my position as a Commanding Officer of a Naval Security Forces reserve unit at NAS Fallon because of the LAPD. I've lost a relationship with my mother and sister because of the LAPD. I've lost a relationship with close friends because of the LAPD. In essence, I've lost everything because the LAPD took my name when they knew I was INNOCENT!!!

XXXX, XXXX, XXXX, and XXXX all knew I was innocent but decided to terminate me so they could retain Officer XXXX. I know about the meeting between all of you where XXXX's attorney, XXXX, confessed that she had kicked XXXX with excessive force. Your day has come.

I'm not an aspiring rapper, I'm not a gang member, I'm not a dope dealer, and I don't have multiple baby mommas. I am an American by choice, I am a son, I am a brother, I am a military service member, and I am a man who lost complete faith in the system when that system betrayed, slandered, and libeled me.

I lived a good life, and though I'm not a religious man I always stuck to my own personal code of ethics, ethos, and my shoreline and true North. I didn't need the US Navy to instill in me Honor, Courage, and Commitment, but I thank them for reinforcing it. It's in my DNA.

Luckily, I don't have to live everyday like most of you. You'll always be worried that the misconduct you were a part of is going to be discovered, constantly looking over your shoulder, scurrying at every phone call from internal affairs or from the Captains office wondering if this is the day PSB comes after you for the suspects you struck when they were cuffed months and years ago, or for that $500 you pocketed from the narcotics dealer, or for when the other guys on your watch beat a transient nearly to death and you never reported the UOF to the supervisor.

No, I don't have that concern. I stood up for what was right, but unfortunately have dealt with the repercussions of doing the right thing—losing my name and everything I ever stood for. You fuckers knew XXXX was guilty of kicking XXXX (with excessive force) and you did nothing but get rid of what you saw as the problem: the whistleblower. XXXX himself stated on video (provided for the BOR and in transcripts) that he was kicked, and even his father stated that his son said he was kicked by XXXX upon release from custody. The video was played for the entire BOR to hear. You're going to see what a whistleblower can do when you take everything away from him, especially his NAME!!!

Look what you did to Sergeant XXXX (now lieutenant) when he exposed the truth of your lying, racism, and PSB cover-ups to frame and convict an innocent man. You cannot police yourselves, and implementing the consent decree was unsuccessful. Sergeant XXXX, I met you on the range several times as a recruit and as an officer. You're a good man and I saw it in your eyes and through your actions.

Self-preservation is no longer important to me. I do not fear death, as I died long ago on Jan. 2, 2009. I was told by my mother that sometimes bad things happen to good people. I refuse to accept that.

From February 2005 to January 2009 I saw some of the most vile things humans can do to each other as a police officer in Los Angeles. Unfortunately, it wasn't in the streets of LA. It was in the confines of LAPD police stations and shops (cruisers). The enemy combatants in LA are not the citizens and suspects, they're the police officers.

People who live in glass houses should not throw stones. How ironic, then, that you utilize a fixed glass structure as your command HQ. You sit in a luminous building to symbolize that you are transparent and have nothing to hide or suppress when in essence, concealing, omitting, and obscuring are your forte.

Chief Beck, this is when you need to have that "come to Jesus" talk with Sergeant XXXX and everyone else who was involved in the conspiracy to have me terminated for doing the right thing. You also need to speak with XXXX's attorney, Rico, about his conversation with the BOR members and her confession of guilt in kicking Mr. XXXX. I'll be waiting for a PUBLIC response at a press conference. When the truth comes out, the killing stops.

Why didn't you charge me with filing a false police report when I came forward stating that XXXX kicked Mr. XXXX? You file criminal charges against every other officer who is accused and terminated for filing a false police report. You didn't charge me because you knew I was innocent and a criminal court would find me so, exposing your department for suppressing the truth and retaliation, that's why.

The attacks will stop when the department states the truth about my innocence, PUBLICLY!!! I will not accept any type of currency/goods in exchange for the attacks to stop, nor do I want any. I want my name back, period. There is no negotiation. I am not the State Department who merely states they do not negotiate with terrorist, because anyone with a Secret or TS/SCI has seen IIR's on SIPR and knows that the US State Department always negotiates by using CF countries or independent sovereign/neutral country to mediate and compromise.

This department has not changed from the Daryl Gates and Mark Fuhrman days. Those officers are still employed and have all been promoted to Command staff and supervisory positions. I will correct this error. Are you aware that an officer (a rookie/probationer at the time) seen on the Rodney King videotape striking Mr. King multiple times with a baton on March 3, 1991 is still employed by the LAPD and is now a Captain in the police department? Captain XXXX is now the commanding officer of a LAPD police station (West LA Division).

As a commanding officer, he is now responsible for over 200 officers. Do you trust him to enforce department policy and investigate use of force investigations on arrestees by his officers? Are you aware XXXX has since been promoted to Sergeant after kicking Mr. XXXX in the face? Oh, you violated a citizen's civil rights? We will promote you. The same as LAPD did with the officers from Metro involved in the May Day melee at MacArthur Park. They were promoted to Sergeant (a supervisor role).

No one is saying you can't be prejudiced or a bigot. We are all human and hold prejudices. If you state that you don't have prejudices, you're lying! But, when you act on it and victimize innocent citizens and fellow innocent officers, then that is a concern.

For the officers who do the job in the name of JUSTICE, those of you who lost honest officers to this event, look at the name of those on the BOR and the investigating officers from PSB and XXXX and ask them, how come you couldn't tell the truth? Why did you terminate an honest officer and cover for a dishonest officer who victimized a mentally ill citizen?

Sometimes humans feel a need to prove they are the dominant race, and they inadvertently take kindness for weakness from another individual. You chose wrong.

Terminating officers because they expose a culture of lying, racism (from the academy), and excessive use of force will immediately change. PSB cannot police their own, and that has been proven. The blue line will forever be severed and a cultural change will be implanted. You have awoken a sleeping giant.

I am here to change and make policy. The culture of the LAPD towards the community and honest, good officers needs to and will change. I am here to correct and calibrate your morale compasses to true north.

To those Caucasian officers who join South Bureau Divisions (77th, SW, SE, and Harbor) with the sole intent to victimize minorities who are uneducated, unaware of criminal law, civil law, and civil rights: you prefer the South Bureau because a use of force/deadly force is likely, and the individual you use UOF on will likely not report it. You are a high value target.

To those Black officers in supervisory ranks and pay grades who stay in South Bureau (even though you live in the valley or OC) for the sole intent of getting retribution on subordinate Caucasian officers for the pain and hostile work environment their elders inflicted on you as probationers (P-1's) and novice P-2's: You are a high value target. You perpetuated the cycle of racism in the department as well. You breed a new generation of bigoted Caucasian officer when you belittle them and treat them unfairly.

To those Hispanic officers who victimize their own ethnicity because they are new immigrants to this country and are unaware of their civil rights: you call them wetbacks to their face and demean them in front of fellow officers of different ethnicities to gain some sort of acceptance from your colleagues. I'm not impressed. Most likely, your parents or grandparents were immigrants at one time, but you have forgotten that. You are a high value target.

To those lesbian officers in supervising positions who go to work, day in and day out, with the sole intent of attempting to prove your misandrist authority (not feminism) to degrade male officers: You are a high value target.

To those Asian officers who stand by and observe everything I previously mentioned other officers participate in on a daily basis but you say nothing, stand for nothing, and protect nothing: Why? Because of your usual saying, "I . . . don't like conflict." You are a high value target as well.

To those of you who "go along to get along," have no backbone, and destroy the foundation of courage: You are the enablers of those who are guilty of misconduct. You are just as guilty as those who break the code of ethics and oath you swore.

To citizens/non-combatants: do not render medical aid to downed officers/enemy combatants. They would not do the same for you. They will let you bleed out just so they can brag to other officers that they had a 187 caper the other day and can't wait to accrue the overtime in future court subpoenas. As they always say, "that's the paramedics' job . . . not mine." Let the balance of loss of life take place. Sometimes a reset needs to occur.

The number of times per week officers arrest an individual, label him a suspect-arrestee-defendant, and then, before arraignment or trial, realize that he is innocent based on evidence is unending. You know what they say when they realize an innocent man just had his life turned upside down? "I guess he should have stayed at home that day he was discovered walking down the street and matching the suspect's description. Oh well, he appeared to be a dirtbag anyways". Meanwhile the falsely accused is left to pick up his life, get a new family, friends, and sense of self-worth.

Don't honor these fallen officers/dirtbags. When your family members die, they just see you as extra overtime at a crime scene and at a perimeter. Why would you value their lives when they clearly don't value yours or your family members' lives? I've heard many officers who state they see dead victims as ATV's, WaveRunners, RV's, and new clothes for their kids.

Why would you shed a tear for them when they, in return, crack a smile for your loss because of the impending extra money they will receive in their next paycheck for sitting at your loved ones' crime scene for six hours because of the overtime they will accrue? They take photos of your loved ones' recently deceased bodies with their cell phones and play a game to see who has the most graphic dead body of the night with officers from other divisions. This isn't just the 20-something-year-old officers; this is the 50-year-old officers with significant time on the job who participate as well.

You allow an officer, XXXX, that attempts to hack into my credit union account to remain on the job even after Detective XXXX provides evidence that the IP address (provided by LAPFCU) that attempted to hack into my account and change my username and password leads directly to her residence. You even allow this visibly disgusting-looking officer to stay on the job when she perjures (lies) herself in court (Clark County Family Court) to and denies hacking into my personal credit union online account when I attempted to get my restraining order extended. Detective XXXX provided the evidence and you still do nothing.

How do you know when a police officer is lying??? When he begins his sentence with, "based on my experience and training."

No one grows up and wants to be a cop killer. It was against everything I've ever been about. As a young police explorer I found my calling in life. But, as a young police officer, I found that the violent suspects on the street are not the only people you have to watch. There's also the officer who was hired on to the department (pre-2000) before polygraphs were standard for all new hires, and a substantial vetting and background investigation were in place.

To those children of the officers who are eradicated, your parent was not the individual you thought they were. As you get older, you will see the evidence that your parent was a tyrant who lost their ethos and instead followed the path of moral corruptness. They conspired to hide and suppress the truth of misconduct on others' behalf. Your parent will have a name and plaque on the fallen officers' memorial in D.C. But, in all honesty, your parent's name will be a reminder to other officers to maintain the oath they swore and to stay along the shoreline that has guided them from childhood to that of a local, state, or federal law enforcement officer.

Your lack of ethics and time conspiring to wrong a just individual are over. Suppressing the truth will lead to deadly consequences for you and your family. There will be an element of surprise where you work, live, eat, and sleep. I will utilize ISR at your home, workplace, and all locations in between. I will utilize OSINT to discover your residences, spouse's workplaces, and children's schools. IMINT will coordinate and plan attacks on your fixed locations. It's amazing what's on NIPR. HUMINT will be utilized to collect personal schedules of targets. I never had the opportunity to have a family of my own, so I'm terminating yours. XXXX, XXXX, XXXX, and BOR members, look your wives/husbands and surviving children directly in the face and tell them the truth as to why your children are dead.

Never allow a LAPPL union attorney to be a retired LAPD Captain, XXXX. He doesn't work for you, your interest, or your name. He works for the department, period. His job is to protect the department from civil lawsuits being filed, and his best interest is the almighty dollar. His loyalty is to the department, not his client. Even when he knows you're innocent and the BOR also knows you're innocent, after XXXX stated on videotape that he was kicked and XXXX's attorney confessed to the BOR off the record that she kicked XXXX.

"The tree of liberty must be refreshed from time to time with the blood of patriots and tyrants" – Thomas Jefferson. This quote is not directed toward the US government which I fully support 100%. This is directed toward the LAPD who cannot monitor itself. The consent decree should never have been lifted, ever.

I know your TTP's (techniques, tactics, and procedures). Any threat assessments you generate will be useless. This is simple; I know your TTP's and PPR's. I will mitigate any of your attempts at preservation. ORM is my friend. I will mitigate all risks, threats, and hazards. I assure you that Incident Command Posts will be target rich environments. KMA-367 license plate frames are great target indicators and make target selection even easier.

I will conduct DA operations to destroy, exploit, and seize designated targets. If unsuccessful or unable to meet objectives in these initial small-scale offensive actions, I will reassess my BDA and re-attack until objectives are met. I have nothing to lose. My personal casualty means nothing. Just like AAF's, ACM's, and AIF's, you cannot prevail against an enemy combatant who has no fear of death. An enemy who embraces death is a lose-lose situation for their enemy combatants.

Hopefully you analysts have done your homework. You are aware that I have always been the top shot, highest score, and expert in rifle qualifications in every unit I've been in. I will utilize every bit of small arms training, demolition, ordnance, and survival training I've been given.

Do you know why we are unsuccessful in asymmetrical and guerrilla warfare in CENTCOM theatre of operations? I'll tell you. It's not the inefficiency of our combatant commanders, planning, readiness, or training of troops. Much like the Vietnam War, ACM, AAF, foreign fighters, Jihadist, and JAM have nothing to lose. They embrace death as it is a way of life. I simply don't fear it. I am the walking exigent circumstance you created.

The violence of action will be HIGH. I am the reason TAC alert was established. I will bring unconventional and asymmetrical warfare to those in LAPD uniform whether on-or off-duty. ISR is my strength and your weakness. You will now live the life of the prey.

Your RD's and homes away from work will be my AO and battle space. I will utilize every tool within INT collections that I learned from NMITC in Dam Neck. You have misjudged a sleeping giant. There is no conventional threat assessment for me. JAM, New Ba'ath party, 1920 rev BGE, ACM, AAF, AQAP, AQIM, and AQIZ have nothing on me. Do not deploy airships or gunships. SA-7 Manpads will be waiting. As you know, I also own Barrett .50s so your APC are defunct and futile.

You better have all your officers radio/phone muster (code 1) on- or off-duty every hour, on the hour.

Do not attempt to shadow or conduct any type of ISR on me. I have the inventory listing of all UC vehicles at Piper Tech and the home addresses of any INT analyst at JRIC and detachment locations. My POA is always POI and always true. This will be a war of attrition and a Pyrrhic and Camdean Victory for myself. You may have the resources and manpower, but you are reactive and predictable in your op plans and TTPs. I have the strength and benefits of being unpredictable, unconventional, and unforgiving. Do not waste your time with briefs and tabletops.

Whatever pre-planned responses you have established for a scenario like me, shelve it. Whatever contingency plan you have, shelve it. Whatever tertiary plan you've created, shelve it. I am a walking exigent circumstance with no OFF or reset button. JRIC, DOJ, LASD, FBI, and other local LE can't assist and should not involve themselves in a matter that does not concern them. For all other agencies, do not involve yourselves in this capture or recovery of me. Look at the big picture of the situation. They (LAPD) created the situation. I will harm no outside agency unless it is a deadly force/IDOL situation. With today's budgeting and fiscal mess, you guys cannot afford to lose several officers to IOD or KIA/EOW. Plus, other officers should not have to take on the additional duties and responsibilities of dead officers. Think about their families, outside agencies, and Chiefs/Directors.

To outside agencies and individual officers on patrol: if you recognize my vehicle, and confirm it is my vehicle through a DMV/ want warrant check, it behooves you to respond to dispatch that your query was for information purposes only. If you proceed with a traffic stop, attempt to notify other officers of my location, or radio for backup, you will not live to see the Medal of Valor you were hoping to receive for your actions. Think before you attempt to intervene. You will not survive.

Your family will receive that Medal of Valor posthumously. It will gather dust on the fireplace mantel for years. Then one day, it will go in a shoe box with other memories. Your mother will lose a son or daughter. Your significant other will be left alone, but they will find someone else to fill your void in the future and make them just as happy. Your children, if you have them, will call someone else mommy or daddy. Don't be selfish. Your vest is only a level II or IIIA, think about it.

No amount of IMINT, MASINT, and ELINT will assist you in capturing me. I am off the grid. You better use your feet, tongue, and every available DOD/NON-DOD HUMINT agency and contractor to find me. I know your route to and from home and your division. I know your significant others' routine, your children's best friends, and recess schedule. I know your Sancha's gym hours and routine. I assure you that the casualty rate will be high. Because of that, no one will remember your name. You will merely become a DR# and "that guy" who was KIA/EOW or long term IOD/light duty in the kit room. This is exactly why "station 500" was created.

Unfortunately, orphanages will be making a comeback in the 21st century.

If you had a well regulated AWB, this would not happen. The time is now to reinstitute a ban that will save lives. Why does any sportsman need a 30 round magazine for hunting? Why does anyone need a suppressor? Why does anyone need an AR15 rifle? This is the same small arms weapons system utilized in eradicating Al Qaeda, Taliban, and every enemy combatant since the Vietnam War. Don't give me that crap that it's not a select fire or full-auto rifle like the DOD uses. That's (expletive) because troops who carry the M-4/M-16 weapon system for combat ops outside the wire rarely utilize the select fire function when in contact with enemy combatants. The use of select fire probably isn't even 1% in combat. So, in essence, the AR-15 semiautomatic rifle is the same as the M-4/M-16. These shouldn't be purchased as easily as walking to your local Walmart or striking the enter key on your keyboard to "add to cart." All the firearms utilized in my activities are registered to me and were legally purchased at gun stores and private party transfers. All concealable weapons (pistols) were also legally registered in my name at police stations or FFL's. Unfortunately, are you aware that I obtained class III weapons (suppressors) without a background check through NICS or DROS completely LEGALLY several times? I was able to use a trust account that I created on Quicken WillMaker and a $10 notary charge at a Mail Boxes etc. to obtain them legally. Granted, I am not a felon, nor do I have a DV misdemeanor conviction or active TRO against me on a NCIC file. I can buy any firearm I want, but should I be able to purchase these class III weapons (SBR's, and suppressors) without a background check, and with just a $10 notary signature on a Quicken WillMaker program? The answer is NO. I'm not even a resident of the state I purchased them in. Lock n Load just wanted money so they allow you to purchase class III weapons with just a notarized trust, military ID. Shame on you, Lock n Load. NFA and ATF need new laws and policies that do not allow loopholes such as this. In the end, I hope that you will realize that the small arms I utilize should not be accessed with the ease with which I obtained them. Who in their right mind needs a (expletive) silencer!!! Who needs a freaking SBR AR15? No one. No more Virginia Tech, Columbine HS, Wisconsin temple, Aurora theatre, Portland malls, Tucson rally, Newtown Sandy Hook. Whether by executive order or through a bi-partisan congress, an assault weapons ban needs to be re-instituted. Period!!!

Mia Farrow said it best: "Gun control is no longer debatable, it's not a conversation, its a moral mandate."

Senator Feinstein, you are doing the right thing in leading the re-institution of a national AWB. Never again should any public official state that their prayers and thoughts are with the families of victims. That has become cliché and meaningless. It's time for action. Let this be the legacy that you bestow to America. Do not be swayed by obstacles, antagonists, and naysayers. Remember the innocent children at Austin, Kent, Stockton, Fullerton, San Diego, Iowa City, Jonesboro, Columbine, Nickel Mines, Blacksburg, Springfield, Red Lake, Chardon, Aurora, and Newtown. Make sure this never happens again!!!

In my cache you will find several small arms. In the cache, there are Bushmaster firearms, Remington precision rifles, and AAC Suppressors (silencers). All of these small arms are manufactured by Cerberus/Freedom Group. The same company that is responsible for the Portland mall shooting, Webster, NY, and Sandy Hook massacre.

You disrespect the office of the POTUS/Presidency and Commander in Chief. You call him Kenyan, mongroid, halfrican, Muslim, and FBHO when in essence you are to address him as simply, President. The same as you did to President George W. Bush and all those in the highest ranking position of our land before him. Just as I always have. You question his birth certificate, his educational and professional accomplishments, and his Judeo-Christian beliefs. You make disparaging remarks about his dead parents. You never questioned the fact that his former opponent, the honorable Senator John McCain, was not born in the CONUS or that Bush had a C average in his undergrad. Electoral Candidates' children (Romney) state they want to punch the president in the face during debates with no formal repercussions. No one even questioned the fact that the son just made a criminal threat toward the President. You call his wife a Wookie. Off the record, I love your new bangs, Mrs. Obama. A woman whose professional and educational accomplishments are second to none when compared to recent First Ladies. You call his supporters, whether black, brown, yellow, or white, leeches, FSA, welfare recipients, and [expletive] lovers. You say this openly without any discretion. Before you start with your argument that you believe I would vote for Obama because he has the same skin color as me, [expletive] you. I didn't vote in this last election as my choice of candidate, John Huntsman, didn't win the primary candidacy for his party. Mr. President, I haven't agreed with all of your decisions but of course I haven't agreed with all of your predecessors' decisions. I think you've done a hell of a job with what you have been dealt and how you have managed it. I shed a tear the night you were initially elected President in 2008. I never thought that day would occur. A black man elected president in the U.S. in my lifetime. I cracked a smiled when you were re-elected in 2012 because I really didn't think you were going to pull that one off. Romney, stop being a sore loser. You could've exited graciously and still contributed significantly to public service. Not now. Mr. President, get back to work. Many want to see you fail as they have stated so many times previously. Unfortunately, if you fail, the U.S. fails, but your opponents do not concern themselves with the big picture. Do not forget your commitment to transparency in your administration. Sometimes I believe your administration forgets that. America, you will realize today and tomorrow that this world is made up of all human beings who have the same general needs and wants in life for themselves, their kin, community, and state. That is the freedom to LIVE and LOVE. They may eat different foods, enjoy different music, have different dialects, or speak a second language, but in essence are no different from you or me. This is America. We are not a perfect sovereign country, as we have our own flaws, but we are the closest that will ever exist.

Unfortunately, this is not the first time an authoritative figure has lied to me.

Mr. XX, assistant principal, XX HS. Remember when you lied to my mother and the police officer in your office when you stated that you never told me in a private conversation that you knew the theft suspect (xx) stole my watch? Let me refresh your memory. A physical education teacher's assistant, a student, stole the list of combination codes to peoples' lockers from the P.E. teacher. That student then opened many of those lockers and stole students' personal property. My watch was taken in that multi-theft and I reported it to you. A week later you discovered that the theft suspect was XX XX, a student. You stated to me in private that you knew for a fact that he stole my property. When I attempted to retrieve my property from the suspect, campus security was called and you lied—stating that you never told me that you "know he stole my watch." You sat there and lied to their faces right in front of me. You said it with such a deliberate, stern face. I never forgot that and was not surprised when 13 years later I was lied about again in the BOR by XX XX. Maybe you can confess to your family at the very least in the private of your own home. After that, contact my mother and apologize for lying to her in 1996.

If possible, I want my brain preserved for science/research to study the effects of severe depression on an individual's brain. Since June 26, 2008, when I was relieved of duty, and Jan. 2, 2009, when I was terminated, I have been afflicted with severe depression. I've had two CT scans during my lifetime that are in my medical record at Kaiser Permanente. Both are from concussions resulting from playing football. The first one was in high school, October 1996. The second was in college and occurred in October 1999. Both were conducted at Kaiser Permanente hospitals in LA/Orange County. These two CT scans should give a good baseline for my brain activity before severe depression began in late 2008.

Sure, many of you "law enforcement experts and specialists" will state, "in all my years this is the worst…" Stop!!! That's not important. Ask yourselves what would cause somebody to take these drastic measures as I have. That's what is important.

To my friends listed below, I wish we could have grown old together and spent more time together. When you reminisce of our friendship and experiences, think of that and that only. Do not dwell on my recent actions the last few days. This was a necessary evil that had to be executed in order for me to recover my NAME. The only thing that changes policy and garners attention is death.

XX XX, greatest friend, Marine officer, aviator, and an even better father and husband. I couldn't have had a better big brother than you. I always cherished your spoken wisdom, you old salty Mustang. You sternly told me that no matter what I accomplish, I will always be a ni#%er in many individuals' eyes. At the time, I did not comprehend your words. I do now. I never forgot the quote you said below. I love you bro.

"I never saw a wild thing feel sorry for itself. A small bird will drop frozen dead from a bough without ever feeling sorry for itself." D.H. Lawrence

XX XX, greatest friend, Naval officer, aviator, great father, husband, doctor, and even better human being. I always strived to live my life parallel to yours, with similar values and personal disciplines. XX is lucky to have found a man like you, and you are fortunate to have married an irrefutably imperfect woman. Always focus on your IMMEDIATE family, as they are the ones who have loved you unconditionally and always been there to support you in difficult times. I always lived my life as WWJD (what would XX do). XX, take care of this guy. XX, I'm sorry I missed your wedding and you had to find another best man. I'm sorry my predicament with the department stopped me from watching you and XX get married, and for arguing with you about issues that were insignificant when I was really angry at the LAPD for what they did to me. I'm deeply sorry and I love you guys.

XX, great friend, attorney, father, husband, and the most cynical/ blatant/politically incorrect friend a man can have. The best quality about you in college and now is that you never sugarcoated the truth. I will miss our political discussions that always turned into arguments. Thanks for introducing me to outdoor sports like fishing, hunting, mudding, and also respect for the land and resources. Us city boys don't get out much like you Alaskans. You even introduced me to PBR. A beer, that when you're a poor college student, is completely acceptable to get buzzed off of. I'm sorry I'll never get to go on that moose and bear hunt with you. I love you bro.

XX, greatest friend, accountant, entrepreneur, and even better human being. You are probably the most well balanced person I've ever met and the most driven for success. In college, and after graduation, I was inspired by your personal drive. Never settle. When you make your first million, promise me you won't forget to enjoy it a bit. I know your first reaction will be to invest it somewhere else. Spend a little, just a little. I love you bro.

XX XX, great friend, entrepreneur, husband, and father. You showed me the importance of fatherhood and friendship. Love you bro.

[Names redacted]

You guys were all important and very special to me. Don't be angry with me. I missed some of your weddings and unfortunately, some of your funerals. This was a necessary evil.

Some say it is my own fault that I was terminated. Yes, XXX, I remember you telling me this in an angry fit. You said that I should have kept my mouth shut about another officer's misconduct. Maybe you were right. But I'm not built like others, it's not in my DNA, and my history has always shown that. When you view the video of the suspect stating he was kicked by XX, maybe you will see that I was a decent person after all. I told the truth. It still hurt that you abandoned me in my time of need. I hope you're happy, that's all I ever wanted for you.

Sergeant XX XX, you meant well but you should have known from your time on the job that the department would attempt to protect someone like XX because of her time on the job, personal friendships, and ethnicity. I'm not angry with you, but you should have known as an IA investigator.

Sergeant XX XX LPPD, Officer XX XX LPPD (ret), and Chief XX XX LPPD, your guidance and mentoring as a young police explorer was second to none and invaluable as a young man, police officer, and Naval officer. Sergeant XX, you forewarned me long ago about joining LAPD as they were "different" and operated differently from other modern law enforcement agencies. I now know it was your humbleness and respect for all who wear the badge and protect their communities that you didn't just express what you wanted to say, that they lack values and basic ethics as law enforcement officers. Chief XX, your (expletive) awesome. Thanks for the long talks over the years when I was an explorer, college student, Naval officer, and police officer. You are a great leader and carry your heart on your sleeve. Your son will be a great Air Force officer with the upbringing you provided. XX, what can I say? You're just an awesome person and my first exposure to what law enforcement was really about was on our ride-alongs. Your realistic approach and empathetic approach to treating all people as humans first is something I carried with me daily. Thank you, every one of you.

Dr. XX, thank you for the superb surgery you performed on my knee in July 1998 in Irvine, Calif. I never had the opportunity to thank you for allowing me to live a life free of knee joint pain. Thank you.

CM1 XX (Ret.), I learned more from you about leadership than most of my own commanders. You lived by a strict ethos of get it done, and get it done right. I wanted to attend your retirement, I really did. But because of my predicament I was unable to. Hope you and XX are still together. I've always held you in high regard.

Sergeant Major XX "XX" XX USMC, Thank you for the intense instruction, mentorship, and time spent forging me into a never-quit officer. You were challenging as a DI. You made sure the vicious and intense personality I possess was discovered. On a lighter note… Don't feel humbled you never broke me. I made it a personal goal to never give up years before. The Corp is lucky to have you at the front. Your leadership is essential and needed for all Marines, especially staff NCO's and mentorship and advisement to company grade officers. You are the epitome of a US Marine and never forget that.

I thank my friends for the awesome shared experiences. I thank the unnamed women I dated over my lifetime for the great and sometimes not so great sex.

It's kind of sad I won't be around to view and enjoy The Hangover III. What an awesome trilogy. XX XX, don't make anymore Hangovers after the third; it takes away the originality of its foundation. World War Z looks good and The Walking Dead season 3 (second half) looked intriguing. Damn, gonna miss Shark Week.

Mr. Vice President, do your due diligence when formulating a concise and permanent national AWB plan. Future generations of Americans depend on your plan and advisement to the president. I've always been a fan of yours and consider you one of the few genuine and charismatic politicians. Damn, sounds like an oxymoron calling you an honest politician. It's the truth.

Hillary Clinton. You'll make one hell of a president in 2016. Much like your husband, Bill, you will be one of the greatest. Look to Castro in San Antonio as a running mate or possible Secretary of State. He's (good people) and I have faith and confidence in him. Look after Bill. He was always my favorite President.

Chelsea grew up to be one hell of an attractive woman. No disrespect to her husband.

Governor Chris Christie. What can I say? You're the only person I would like to see in the White House in 2016 other than Hillary. You're America's no (expletive) taking uncle. Do one thing for your wife, kids, and supporters. Start walking at night and eat a little less, not a lot less, just a little. We want to see you around for a long time. Your leadership is greatly needed.

Wayne LaPierre, President of the NRA, you're a vile and inhumane piece of (expletive). You never even showed 30 seconds of empathy for the children, teachers, and families of Sandy Hook. You deflected any type of blame/responsibility and directed it toward the influence of movies and the media. You are a failure of a human being. May all of your immediate and distant family die horrific deaths in front of you.

Chris Matthews, Joe Scarborough, Pat Harvey, Brian Williams, Soledad Obrien, Wolf Blitzer, Meredith Viera, Tavis Smiley, and Anderson Cooper, keep up the great work and follow Cronkite's lead. I hold many of you in the same regard as Tom Brokaw and the late Peter Jennings. Cooper, stop nagging and berating your guests, they're your (guests). Mr. Scarborough, we met at McGuire's pub in P-cola in 2002 when I was stationed there. It was an honor conversing with you about politics, family, and life.

Willie Geist, you're a talented and charismatic journalist. Stop with all the talk show shenanigans and get back to your core of reporting. Your future is brighter than most.

Revoke the citizenship of Fareed Zakaria and deport him. I've never heard a positive word about America or its interests from his mouth, ever. On the same day, give Piers Morgan an indefinite resident alien and Visa card. Mr. Morgan, the problem that many American gun owners have with you and your continuous discussion of gun control is that you are not an American citizen and have an accent that is distinct and clarifies that you are a foreigner. I want you to know that I agree with you 100% on enacting stricter firearm laws but you must understand that your critics will always have in the back of their mind that you are native to a country that we won our sovereignty from while using firearms as a last resort, and you come from a country that has no legal private ownership of firearms. That is disheartening to American gun owners and rightfully so.

The honorable President George H.W. Bush, they never give you enough credit for your successful presidency. You were always one of my favorite presidents (2nd favorite). I hope your health improves greatly. You are the epitome of an American and provided a great service to your country.

General Petraeus, you made a mistake that the majority of men make once, twice, or unfortunately many times in a lifetime. You are human. You thought with your penis. It's okay. I personally believe you should have never resigned and told your critics to shove it. You only answer to two people regarding the affair: your wife and children, period. I hope you return to government service for your country as it is visibly in your DNA.

General Colin Powell, your book "My American Journey" solidified my decision to join the military after college. I had always intended to serve, but your book and journey motivated me. You are an inspiration to all Americans and influenced me greatly.

To all SEA's (senior enlisted advisers), you are just as important, if not more so, in the viability of large and small commands. It's time you take a more active role in leading your enlisted and advising officers. These are not your twilight years or time to relax. You can either strengthen the tip of the spear, or make it brittle.

You decide.

Pat Harvey, I've always thought you carried yourself, professionally and personally, the way a strong black woman should. Your articulation and speech is second to none. You are the epitome of a journalist/anchor. You are America.

Ellen DeGeneres, continue your excellent contribution to entertaining America and bringing the human factor to entertainment. You changed the perception of your gay community and how we as Americans view the LGBT community. I congratulate you on your success and opening my eyes as a young adult, and my generation to the fact that you are no different from us other than who you choose to love. Oh, and you Prop 8 supporters, why the (expletive) do you care who your neighbor marries? Hypocritical pieces of (expletive).

Westboro Baptist Church, may you all burn slowly in a fire, not from smoke inhalation, but from the flames and only the flames.

Tebow, I really wanted to see you take charge of the game and an offense again. You are not a good QB by today's standards, but you are a great football player who knows how to lead a team and WIN. You will be "Tebowing" when you reach your next team. I have faith in you. Get out of that circus they call the Jets and away from the reality TV star, Rex Ryan, and Mark Rapist Sanchez.

Christopher Walz, you impressed me in Inglorious Basterds. After viewing Django Unchained, I was sold. I have come to the conclusion that you are well on your way to becoming one of the greats, if not already, and show glimpses of Daniel Day Lewis and Morgan Freeman-esque type qualities of greatness. Trust me when I say that you will be one of the greatest ever.

Jennifer Beals, Serena Williams, Grae Drake, Lisa Nicole-Carson, Diana Taurasi, N'bushe Wright, Brenda Villa, Kate Winslet, Ashley Graham, Erika Christensen, Gabrielle Union, Isabella Soprano, Zain Verjee, Tamron Hall, Gina Carano, America Ferrara, Giana Michaels, Nene, Natalie Portman, Queen Latifah, Michelle Rodriguez, Anjelah Johnson, Kelly Clarkson, Nora Jones, Laura Prepon, Margaret Cho, and Rutina Wesley, you are THE MOST beautiful women on this planet, period. Never settle, professionally or personally.

Dave Brubeck's "Take Five" is the greatest piece of music ever, period. Hanz Zimmer, William Bell, Eric Clapton, BB King, Bob Marley, Sam Cooke, Metallica, Rob Zombie, Nora Jones, Marvin Gaye, Jay-Z, and the King (Louis Armstrong) are musical prodigies.

Jeffrey Toobin and David Gergen, you are political geniuses and modern scholars. Hopefully Toobin is nominated for the Supreme Court and implements some damn common sense and reasoning instead of partisan bickering. But in true Toobin fashion, we all know he would not accept the nomination.

John and Ken from KFI, never mute your facts and personal opinions. You are one of the few media personalities who speak the truth, even when the truth is not popular. I will miss listening to your discussions.

Bill Handel, your effin awesome. For years I enjoyed your show.

Anthony Bourdain, you're a modern renaissance man who epitomizes the saying "too cool for school".

Larry David, Kevin Hart, the late Patrice O'Neal, Lisa Lampanelli, Chris Rock, Jerry Seinfeld, Louis CK, Dave Chapelle, Jon Stewart, Wanda Sykes, Dennis Miller, and Jeff Ross are pure geniuses. I'm a big fan of all of your work. As a child, my mom caught me watching Def Jam comedy at midnight when I should have been asleep. Instead of scolding me, the next night she let me stay up late and watch

George Carlin, Eddie Murphy, and Richard Pryor comedy specials with her for hours. My sides were sore for days.

Larry David, I agree. 72-82 degrees is way too hot in a residence. 68 degrees is perfect.

Cyclists, I have no problem sharing the road with you. But, at least go the (expletive) speed limit posted or get off the road!!! That is a fair request.

Livestrong you fraudulent (expletive).

Cardinal Mahoney, you are in essence a predator yourself as you enabled your subordinates to molest multiple children in the church over many decades.

May you die a long and slow, painful death.

If you continuously followed me while I was walking at dusk/night I would confront you as well. Too bad Trayvon didn't smash your skull completely open, Zim. While Trayvon's body erodes to bones 6 feet under, Zimmerman has put on no less than 40 pounds while out on bail. Zimmerman was arrested for battery on a Peace officer and avoided jail/prison because he completed a diversion program. That's a history of being an (expletive). Zimmerman couldn't get hired by a LE agency because of poor credit/and a history of violence/restraining orders with women. So what does he do? Designate himself neighborhood watch captain and make complaints to his city council about the horrible work ethic and laziness of the officers patrolling his neighborhood. Good one Zim.

How classy that your father attempts to use his veteran's status, "disabled veteran," during your bail hearing but doesn't state what his disability percentage is.

Prior service personnel know it can be 5% disability to 100%. You and your attorneys always avoid mentioning your father's occupation as a magistrate/judge because I'm sure he's utilized his position to get you out of way more jams than the public has discovered, and that your family is not indigent. Oh, tell your wife to stop perjuring herself in court.

KCCO

Anonymous, you are hated, vilified, and considered an enemy to the state. I personally view you as a culture and a necessity that brings truth to a cloaked world. Forge ahead!

Charlie Sheen, you're effin awesome.

My opinion on women in combat MOS, Designators, Rates, and AFSC's: I wish all of you who attempt to pursue combat occupational roles the greatest success in completing, graduating, and qualifying in your respective schools/courses. Many want to see you fail. Remember, every one of you is a pioneer.

There was a time when they didn't allow blacks to fight the good fight. This is your civil rights. Don't quit!!!

It's time to allow gay service members' spouses to utilize the same benefits that all heterosexual dependents are eligible for. Medical, Dental, Tricare, Deers, SGLI, BX, Commissary, Milstar, MWR, etc. Flag officers, let's be honest. You can't really give a valid argument to as why gays shouldn't be eligible, since every month a new state enacts laws that allow same sex marriage.

To the LGBT community and supporters, the same way you have the right to voice your opinion on acceptance of gay marriage, Chick Fil-A has a right to voice their beliefs as well. That's what makes America so great. Freedom of expression. Don't be (expletive) and boycott/degrade their business and customers who patronize the locations. They make some damn good chicken! Vandalizing (graffiti) their locations does not help any cause.

Mr. Bill Cosby, you are a reasonable and talented man who has spoken the truth of the cultural anomalies within the black communities that need to change now. The black communities' resentment toward you is because they don't like hearing the truth or having their clear and evident dirty laundry aired to the nation. The problem is, the country is not blind or dumb. They believe we are animals. Do not mute your unvarnished, truthful speech or moral compass.

Blacks must strive for more in life than bling, hoes, and cars. The current culture is an epidemic that leaves them with no discernible future. They're suffocating and don't even know it. MLK Jr. would be mortified at what he worked so hard for in gaining acceptance as equal beings, and how, unfortunately, we stopped progressing and began regressing. Chicago's youth violence is a prime example of how our black communities' values have declined. We cannot address this nation's intolerant issues until we address our own communities' morality issues first. Accountability. We need to hold out.

The self-described manifesto ends. However, even a layperson reading this post can sense that Dorner seems rational in his likes and dislikes, even if the totality of them seem like a rant—or, in technical terms, a manic flight of ideas. He says he is trying to clear his name but focuses mostly on not only revenge, but seems to be writing a farewell, a send-off to himself with testimonials to those he admires. It is the ramblings of an insane mind clothed in the trappings of logic and rationality and laden with remorse for a life that failed. But the threats, the dire warnings of catastrophe for those who, he believes, stood against him are in stark menacing contrast to those he praises.

We can ask whether there was any chance of intervening in Dorner's life so as to have avoided any of the chaos he caused. Four lives lost, an engaged couple offered up as a sacrificial revenge against the police captain who defended him at his LAPD hearing, sheriff's officers from Riverside and San Bernadino counties who were ambushed or outgunned by Dorner, and the destruction of property in a manhunt that cost local authorities well into the six figures. Was there a point before all of this started when someone could have defused what, according to friends and intimates, had become a ticking time bomb?

The record indicates that when Dorner had returned to the LAPD in 2007 from his deployment to the Middle East as a Naval reservist, he begged his training officer Sergeant Teresa Evans, for "reintegration" training, which meant that, before going back on patrol in a black and white unit, he would be returned to the LAPD Academy to reacclimate himself to civilian life. Dorner had been an undersea demolitions expert during his service in Bahrain and earned a campaign ribbon for his service in the Iraq War. In the patrol car, according to Sergeant Evans, Dorner actually broke down into tears as he begged for reintegration. Sergeant Evans revealed that Dorner told her he might have had lingering issues regarding his deployment. This is a very important comment, indicating that Dorner was not only having a problem readjusting to civilian law enforcement but that whatever he confronted, or confronted him, during his tour of duty in the Middle East, was eating away at him emotionally. It was a clear and present sign of danger that the LAPD did not respond to.

Sergeant Evans did not send Dorner back to the Academy. Rather, she wrote a negative review of her trainee. The following day, Dorner reported to LAPD's Internal Affairs that he had witnessed Evans assault a mentally ill suspect, a charge that the suspect did not report and which witnesses to the arrest could not corroborate. Dorner was relieved from duty in September, 2008, and fired from the department after a hearing in 2009. After his lawsuit was dismissed by Los Angeles Superior Court in 2011, he filed appeals, all of which were denied. Absent his job, his military career, which formally ended on February 1, 2013, his wife, his fiancée, and everything he used to bolster his own identity, Dorner was alone and awash in hopelessness. A former girlfriend who had shared an apartment with him thought that maybe it was his formal discharge, the end of his military career, that had set him off. By February 3, Dorner was on the move and seeking the revenge of someone casting himself in the role of a commando. Dorner's case, specifically his breakdown in a police unit when he begged Sergeant Evans for help, is a classic example of a military veteran in a decomposing mental state, whether suffering from PTSD or another form of mental illness, sending out a clear signal that something is wrong and being denied help.

We link the Dorner/LAPD case to his service in the military because Dorner blamed his separation from the Navy specifically upon his firing by the LAPD. Thus, one injustice, in his mind, spurred the collapse of his military career, another injustice. If this is an indicator that we expect to see thousands of times over as veterans return from the Middle Eastern wars, then the Dorner case established a proto-pattern. And if the LAPD's response is any indicator, we will have major problems when a sizable number of these returning warriors become pseudo-commandos because they can get no help for invisible wounds of war. According to an article by Dr. James L. Knoll IV in *Psychiatric Times*,[9] the pseudo commando comes laden with sufficient weapons and ammunition to kill indiscriminately as many people as he can, in public, and often in the daytime so his actions will catch more attention. He is prepared to die in a final apocalyptic blaze of glory as if his death is the fitting climax to the destruction he has wrought even while denying authorities the ability to humiliate him by putting him on trial. The pseudocommando is suicidal in that respect, using the instrumentality of his violence to effect that suicide so that his crimes and his death are burned into the public consciousness. At the core of the pseudocommando's suicidal intent is his public statement of self immolation, his act of suicide as revenge against those who have wronged him, and, in so doing, wronged others like him. Thus, Christopher Dorner in his Facebook manifesto characterizes himself as a righteous avenger striking back at those who wronged him, but clothing his actions in righting societal wrongs as well as wrongs done to him. He is fighting racism. He is killing to avenge the lies told about him by the LAPD. He is holding up citizens he believes are models because they, too, are in his mind commandos

---

[9] "The Pseudocommando: Mass Murderer: A Blaze of Vainglory," January 4, 2012

in their own ways. General Colin Powell, Hillary Clinton, and even Charlie Sheen get the nod from Dorner because each, in his or her own way, acts like a righteous commando.

Cho Seung-Hui in his manifesto to NBC News characterized himself as a victim, a Jesus-like figure whose death amidst the deaths of those around him would serve as a form of official notice to all who would bully, ostracize, and victimize people like Cho. And much the same can be said about Norway mass killer Anders Brevik, Texas Tower sniper Charles Whitman, and even Sandy Hook shooter Adam Lanza, all of whom claim to have been seeking to avenge something. When all hope is lost, all avenues closed, the pseudocommando, blaming his target oppressors for his misfortune, makes his final stand taking as many of those oppressors with him to the grave, all of whom are likely completely innocent of the offenses the pseudocommando believes by which he was victimized. Dorner is one of our prime examples of this when it comes to issues arising from military experiences as well as from experiences of those in public safety.

The irony of crimes committed by pseudocommandos is that even though crime and murder rates are dropping nationwide, except for certain areas like Chicago, the amount of casualties created by a suicidal mass murderer, a pseudocommando, seems to defy national crime rates. In fact, as we learn from the recent USA Today research, suicidal mass murders committed by self-styled avenging pseudo commandos is actually on the rise. It is, as we pointed out above, an epidemic.

Chapter 4

Staff Sergeant Robert Bales and the Massacre in Afghanistan

The Afghan National Army sentry at Camp Belambay must have thought it strange when the American staff sergeant stumbled past him well before sunrise on March 11, 2012, and made his way off the base, disappearing into the darkness. Perhaps he was on a mission. Did another sentry also think it strange when the American sergeant returned, still carrying his weapon, and then left the base again? What neither sentry knew was that the American sergeant, Robert Bales, was on a mission, a personal one, during which he killed sixteen Afghan civilians as they slept in their houses, thus setting into motion one of the atrocity scandals of the war in Afghanistan, and perhaps even altering American policy by precipitating an early withdrawal from the combat theater.

Like many patriotic Americans, Robert Bales, who worked as a financial advisor in Ohio, saw the September 11th terrorist attack on the World Trade Center as a defining moment. And, like many patriotic Americans, Bales enlisted in the military, because he saw it as his duty to defend the United States in what President George W. Bush had described as the new War on Terror. He enlisted in November 2001, and had evidently set his mind to do his part and go to war. But those initial powerful feelings of wanting to do something to right the wrongs of September 11th, although heartfelt and legitimate, apparently had begun to sour as Bales slogged his way through multiple contiguous deployments in Iraq and Afghanistan, even after sustaining several injuries.

According to the Army's charge sheet alleging that Staff Sergeant Robert Bales committed premeditated murders of sixteen Afghan civilians—nine of them children—early in the predawn hours of March 11, 2012, Bales left his base, Camp Belambay, in a rural area of southern Afghanistan known as the Panjiway district, and armed with automatic weapons and a knife or other bladed weapon, made his way over a mile on foot under the cover of darkness to a village south of Belambay. Bales did not have permission to leave the base that morning, though he must have walked past at least one Afghan soldier who was guarding the base that night. He was, in effect, absent without leave during the time he was committing the acts for which he is accused.

From the military prosecutor's official charge sheet, it seems that Bales knew where he was going. Once in the quiet village south of his base, the thirty-eight-year-old infantry leader approached the first house, broke in, and while the inhabitants were still asleep, opened fire, killing his victims. Bales left the house and moved on to the next, repeating the same procedure, opening fire and killing the inhabitants. He was stealthy, however, choosing to stab some of the victims quietly in a few of the houses, perhaps to avoid waking the other members of the family. He did not spare women or children as he killed his way from house to house, setting some of the dwellings and bodies on fire, methodically continuing his rampage until all in the village were killed or wounded. No one confronted him.

According to the official accounts of what happened next that morning, Sergeant Bales walked back to his base, again passing an Afghan military guard, waited for an unspecified period of time, during which he allegedly told another American soldier what he had done, and then left his base again to walk to the next neighboring village, this one north of the firebase. The residents there were asleep as well, unaware of the devastation their neighbors had suffered. And just as he had done the first time, according to the Army's same charge sheet, Bales moved from house to house, taking aim and firing at the sleeping families, alternately stabbing some of his victims, until he had inflicted death or critical wounds on all of them. Some of the children hid in fear as they heard the rounds whizzing over their heads, or as the strange man in battlefield khaki attacked their parents with his knife. Very few survived.

Finally the killing was done, and the smoke began to dissipate from the small rooms where bodies lay awash in their own blood. But Bales didn't stay around to survey the damage. Whatever statement he thought he had made, whatever voices he might have been hearing, whatever fury he was wreaking on the civilians from whose villages enemy fire had come and killed members of his unit, or whatever psychological expiation he was seeking from this rampage, Bales was done. The decorated Army sergeant who had suffered brain trauma, partial dismemberment of his foot, and prided himself on his scrupulous behavior discriminating civilians from combatants during his tour of duty in Iraq, now stumbled the mile and a half back towards his base, where, after falling into a ditch, he slept for a while before awakening with an eerie calmness and allegedly turning himself in to authorities. They were waiting for him, having seen a lone soldier on a surveillance video lying face-down on the ground. Staff Sergeant Bales was relieved of his weapon and taken into custody. The soldier he had told about the killings when he returned to the base the first time, between shooting sprees, later said that he didn't believe Bales's story, and therefore, didn't report it. Perhaps the command at Camp Belambay didn't believe at first what had happened, but the news slowly leaked out, and within hours, the true horror of what he had done began to unfold. Bales's civilian defense attorney John Henry Browne, for the record, said that his client never confessed to the killings.

As the story of the murder of Afghani civilians spread across the Internet and through the twenty-four-hour news cycle, the scrutiny began as commentators asked why it had happened, and media-approved, self-described pundit-experts tried to answer the question. However, the real issue of what motivated Staff Sergeant Robert Bales to leave his fire base on March 11 and go on a killing spree may lie deep in the sergeant's domestic background, military history, wounds and brain trauma, hopeless despair and rage at multiple deployments—especially when he believed that he would be promoted to sergeant first class or reassigned stateside as an Army recruiter—or the actual combat mission he believed he was on. Were Bales's actions the result of a complete mental breakdown? Was he striking back against the war itself to find a way out, or something deeper and darker, because he had been assigned as force protection for a Special Forces unit? Was he attempting suicide by proxy; death at the hands of the Taliban in villages where they were allegedly sequestered among the civilian residents? Two of these civilians, who were official witnesses, have already been killed by NATO forces as enemy combatants. Although the answers to these questions might be a long time in coming, they certainly begin with the question of who Robert Bales is, and why he engaged in that killing spree.

One of the first questions that arose as the story of the killings began to spread was, how was it possible for an American soldier to walk off his base without being stopped? Weren't there U.S. troops guarding the facility, and shouldn't they have asked if there was authorization for a soldier to leave the base? The answers quickly emerged that the platoon-sized unit at Camp Belambay was relatively small, perhaps as few as twenty-five soldiers. Guarding the base on the night of March 11 was the responsibility of an American-trained Afghan soldier, part of the Afghan National Army, who did not challenge Bales as he left. Upon his return, another Afghan sentry did not challenge him. Nor was he challenged again upon his second departure. Thus, Bales was able to walk past his guards. It was only when the Afghan sentry notified his officers that an American soldier had left the base that a search was launched for Bales.

According to a *New York Times* description of what happened after the American base command had become aware of the missing soldier, they ordered a search of the entire facility, including the sleeping quarters, food preparation area, and latrines. It was only after the soldier did not turn up that a patrol was organized to search for the missing trooper. However, before the patrol left the base, a surveillance blimp carrying an infrared camera, one of the methods of surveilling the area surrounding the base, was capturing an image of a soldier lying face-down in a nearby field. Infrared cameras capture images by measuring the heat signature emanating from objects the camera is focused on and displaying them against the background of ambient heat. As commanders watched, the soldier got to his feet and began walking back to the base. It was Staff Sergeant Robert Bales.

For some reason, probably because the platoon had so few soldiers, the surveillance camera from the blimp wasn't monitored constantly, and therefore, the image of a soldier walking through the field away from the base wasn't noticed. It was only after the base had become alerted by the Afghan officers that U.S. military personnel checked the monitor carrying the surveillance imagery to search for anyone outside the base perimeter.

When Sergeant Bales returned to the base, his commanders were ready and ordered that the sergeant be disarmed and taken into custody. Perhaps it was only then that the American soldier in whom Bales had confided after the initial shooting spree repeated to officers what Bales had told him, explained that he thought Bales was joking at first, and used that as his reason for not reporting it earlier. Bales was placed under arrest, the immediate issue of how to handle the mass shootings of unarmed civilians confronted his superior officers, and the realization emerged that Bales would be an object of vengeance on the part of the Afghans, possibly the very Afghan troops assigned to Camp Belambay. The Army made an immediate decision, therefore, to get him out of the country and into a safe facility for incarceration as they assessed the evidence for Bales's Article 32 hearing, a preliminary military court appearance to assemble the evidence based on the official charge sheet. And, amidst the new tensions between the Afghan government and the United States, that's how the investigation began.

Had Bales not been a soldier on active duty, and simply perpetrated a mass homicide as a civilian in the United States, his civilian attorney—as did Jared Loughner's attorney after the Tucson, Arizona, mass shooting and multiple homicides—would seek court rulings to determine whether the defendant was competent to stand trial and a psychiatric evaluation to determine whether counsel could raise insanity as an affirmative defense. A person who is judged to be insane is determined not to possess the mental capacity to understand the crime, to differentiate right from wrong, or to comport his behavior to the law because of a mental illness. In order for the prosecution to prove every element of a crime beyond a reasonable doubt— which means that an alternative reasonable explanation that would exonerate the defendant cannot be found—the prosecution must prove that a defendant had formed the mental state—his intent—to commit the crime, and that the defendant, acting upon that mental state, did actually commit the crime. In an insanity defense, the defendant, while admitting to the act, asserts that because of insanity, he was incapable of forming the mental intent to commit the crime. This is how a civilian defense attorney might plead a case like Jared Loughner, or Aurora shooter James Holmes.

However, in the case of Robert Bales, a whole host of other issues arose because he was in the military, on active duty in a combat zone, assigned to a combat base where he was providing protection to a Special Operations Forces unit training local Afghan forces, and therefore, operating as if he were fit for duty. That, in itself, unless a defense can show that he cracked under pressure, presumes he was not insane. Therefore, Bales's background, his prior deployments, his prior combat injuries—including his subconcussive brain trauma—his financial woes back home, and his feelings of hopelessness at having been deployed to Afghanistan after having been promised that he would remain stateside, probably as an Army recruiting sergeant, will all play into the case that will unfold in a military court. Bales likely felt an intense sense of betrayal or even a subtle paranoia that the army was trying to get him killed. This was not a secure setting for a combat veteran believing he was "getting short." In fact, he was not getting short.

Will the defense be able to show that Bales was suffering from Post-Traumatic Stress Disorder to such a degree that it had metastasized into a mental illness that destroyed his rational ability, obliterated his judgment, and made him unfit for duty? Was Bales operating under secret orders that required him to assassinate possible Taliban fighters hiding in the village or protected by its inhabitants? Did Bales see this as his only way out of a hopeless situation in which there was nothing left for him but to die? Or were Bales's actions a new manifestation of My Lai Syndrome, in which frustrated officers, taking fire and losing personnel from what was supposed to be a village of friendlies, finally wreak vengeance? Will defense seek to put the war itself on trial, arguing that, of course, our troops are crumbling under the mental strain of fighting a war that will only end with the withdrawal of those American forces, who only remain in the country to sustain an otherwise corrupt government—installed by the United States—while the remaining troops take fire from the very soldiers they are supposed to be training? And how will a military court handle any exculpatory evidence that may compromise national security? All questions to be asked as the case moves inexorably towards a court martial in a capital crime.

One has to begin with Staff Sergeant Bales's physical and mental condition, as they both apply to Bales's fitness for duty and the objective "fit for duty" standard that governs combat personnel in the field. First, Bales had suffered a combat-related injury in Iraq which resulted in partial amputation of his foot. According to Army regulations, that amputation in itself would have required a reduction in his fitness for duty profile in the orthopedic category. Yet at the time, he was returned to duty after the surgery that removed part of his foot.

Subsequent to his Iraq injury, he was returned to Fort Lewis in Washington State, where his brigade was stationed—a return, after three deployments (one of which was an extended deployment), that he believed would be permanent. He did not think that he would be returned to the front. But Bales had also suffered a concussive brain injury, a head trauma, in Iraq in 2010, which, again, according to the fitness for duty standards, would have reduced his fitness for duty in the neuropsychiatric category. One might conclude, therefore, that a multiplicity of active-duty related injuries would have so reduced his medical fitness rating that a redeployment to an intense battle zone would have been out of the question. Moreover, it has been revealed that at some point, Bales had been taking steroids, a substance that can cause mania even in otherwise healthy people and is prohibited by the Army, and which would have shown up in any blood screening.

There are reports indicating that Bales was also taking an anti-malarial medicine. The Pentagon is in the midst of a widespread review of the military's use of a notorious anti-malaria drug after finding out that the pills have been wrongly given to soldiers with preexisting problems, including brain injuries like the one Bales had sustained. The drug in question, Mefloquine, also called Lariam, has severe psychiatric side effects. Problems include psychotic behavior, paranoia, and hallucinations. The drug has been implicated in numerous suicides and homicides, including deaths in the U.S. military. For years the military has used the weekly pill to help prevent malaria among deployed troops. The U.S. Army nearly dropped use of Mefloquine entirely in 2009 because of the dangers, now only using it in limited circumstances, including sometimes in Afghanistan. The 2009 order from the Army said soldiers who have suffered a traumatic brain injury should not be given the drug. Bales, who suffered a traumatic brain injury in Iraq during his third combat tour, as well as emotional damage during his repeated combat tours, was also a prime risk candidate for the risk of Post-Traumatic Stress Disorder. In 2012, Assistant Secretary of Defense for Health Affairs Jonathan Woodson ordered a review to make sure that troops were not receiving Mefloquine inappropriately. The task order from Woodson begins: "Some deploying service members have been provided Mefloquine for malaria prophylaxis without appropriate documentation in their medical records and without proper screening for contraindications." On March 20, 2012, after the massacre, a follow-up order was sent to the southwest region that says troops in "deployed locations" may be improperly taking the drug.

Army and Pentagon officials would not say whether Bales took the drug, citing privacy rules. When asked if Woodson's Mefloquine review was a response to the massacre, the military in Afghanistan referred the question to the Army, where officials said they were "unaware" of the review. After being shown the task order via email, they stopped responding. The Office of the Secretary of Defense referred questions to the Army, and then back to medical officials in the secretary's office. Those officials have not responded. But the sudden violence and apparent cognitive problems related to the crime Bales is accused of mirrors other gruesome cases.

A former Army psychiatrist who was the top advocate for mental health at the Office of the Army Surgeon General recently voiced concern about Bales's possible Mefloquine exposure. "One obvious question to consider is whether he was on Mefloquine (Lariam), an anti-malarial medication," Dr. Elspeth Cameron Ritchie wrote this week in TIME's *Battleland* blog, noting that the drug, which is associated with certain neuropsychiatric reactions—among which are depression, full-on psychosis, and suicidal ideation—is still used in Afghanistan. In one particular 2010 case, six Army Special Forces members took Mefloquine and committed suicide. Dr. Ritchie has pointed to statistics to argue that suicide is relatively infrequent in Special Forces personnel. One member of the Special Forces described his reaction to the drug by saying that the impulse to hurt yourself or others comes on so suddenly that you don't realize what is happening at first. You just have the urge to commit violence. It should come as no surprise, therefore, that back in 2003, according to the UPI, Mefloquine was related to almost half of the reported suicides in the Army. The following year, when the Army began stopping the use of the drug, suicides dropped by half.

If Bales received Mefloquine, particularly in his at-risk condition, his case may be like Staff Sergeant Georg-Andreas Pogany, whose potential death-sentence charges were dropped by the Army in 2004. Pogany was charged with cowardice, but the Army dropped the charges after doctors determined that Pogany suffered from Lariam toxicity, which affected his behavior in Iraq.

Given his brain trauma and other injuries, not only was Bales deemed to be fit for duty and returned to what he knew to be a remote and dangerous combat assignment, he might also have been given a drug that was known to cause psychotic suicidal and homicidal behavior. His deployment to Afghanistan, yet again, came as a surprise to him—even more of a surprise when he learned that he would be part of a force protection unit assigned to Special Operations Forces.

Among the many issues that seemed to confuse the media regarding Bales's motivations in committing the multiple homicides in Afghanistan was his own statements regarding his role in military combat in Iraq. Bales had been commended by the Army after heavy battles against urban-entrenched hostile forces in Iraq, where part of the challenge was to distinguish the enemy from innocent civilians caught in the cross-fire. This took place during his second deployment at the desperate battle of Najaf, when an Army Apache helicopter crashed and Bales's unit had to fight off over 250 enemy Shiite fighters from the Mahdi militia over a period of two days in order to recover the aircraft. This battle reportedly involved hand-to-hand combat with bayonets.

Bales described the battle as a traditional World War II firefight, in which the American units dug in and eliminated the enemy resistance so as to reach the downed helicopter. In fact, Bales lauded the performance of his unit in Iraq because they withstood enemy fire, returned the fire, routed the enemy, did not incur a single fatality themselves, and accomplished it all while protecting the civilian inhabitants of the area from collateral harm. Moreover, Bales told a newspaper reporter for the *Fort Lewis Northwest Guardian* at Joint Base Fort Lewis-McChord after he returned from his Iraq deployment that after the engagement in which his unit overwhelmed the enemy while protecting civilians, "We helped the very people who, three hours earlier, were trying to kill us." This does not sound like a soldier at the end of his tether who was at risk of taking his rage out on innocent noncombatants. What happened between 2009 and early 2012?

Oddly, although Bales had been wounded in Iraq, he was not awarded a Purple Heart. Moreover, a recommendation for Bales to receive a Bronze Star from the Army was turned down. Other reports suggest that Bales had disciplinary issues with the Army stemming from his questioning orders to return to Afghanistan for a subsequent deployment. Reportedly, Bales had hoped to be sent to either Germany or Italy. He had also been through recruiter training and hoped to become a recruiting sergeant. He reportedly also objected to his orders to return to combat in Afghanistan because of his multiple deployments in Iraq and his belief that his return to Fort Lewis or Europe would be his ultimate destination, where he would serve out the rest of his enlistment. However, his objections were overruled by the Army, and he was reevaluated for medical fitness for duty on the basis of his podiatric injury, which the Army had said was remediated, and the brain trauma that resulted from his blast injury in Iraq.

The neurological imaging that the Army conducted on Bales, which would most likely have been done at Madigan Army Hospital (now at the center of a controversial scandal for falsifying medical records of soldiers), did not show any trauma, according to the medical reports. And Bales was not deemed to be suffering from PTSD, nor did aggression-inciting steroids turn up in his blood.

Criminal charges against Bales were amended by the Army shortly after being filed. The number of homicides he was charged with was reduced by one, from seventeen to sixteen, but the Army added the charge of drinking while on duty. It was reported that on the night of the killings, Bales had been drinking on base—a violation of orders—and might have been taking steroids for the purpose of enhancing performance, building muscle tissue, and improving endurance. Steroids, however, in addition to causing some degree of physical deterioration, can affect people psychologically, altering their moods. It may make them more aggressive, which may cloud or seriously impair judgment and be an incitement to criminal violence. Would it be a defensive strategy to argue for diminished capacity based on the ingestion of substances, which, even though prohibited, might reduce the sentence should Bales be convicted? Would it be a defensive strategy to argue further that, if Bales had been administered antimalarials that are known to cause psychotic and suicidal behavior, and those effects were not known to Bales, might the simple administration of antimalarials be enough to serve as exculpatory evidence, to a degree of diminished capacity, in any capital murder case? It is a point of law that if a person is administered a medication that causes adverse effects to the extent that the effects result in a criminal action, the fact of the administration of that medication may acquit him, or at least have charges against him reduced.

Bales grew up in southern Ohio in the Cincinnati suburb of Norwood, where he was a high school football player and captain of his varsity team. He was popular among his peers and teammates. A former student at Ohio State in Columbus, where he majored in economics, Bales left college to work in the financial services industry and wound up starting a financial consulting business in Florida with his brother. The promise of starting a new company soon turned sour when, because the principals of the company were accused of violating financial service company regulations and were investigated, their license to work in the industry was revoked. Bales never answered the charges brought against him and his colleagues in the company, however, because by the time he was called to testify at a hearing, he had already enlisted in the Army, presumably to start a new career after the September 11th attacks on the World Trade Center.

His enlistment at age twenty-seven, after having started and worked in business, made him a relatively mature enlisted man, immediately more experienced, and probably more of an authority figure. He proved himself both in training and in battle during three deployments in Iraq, serving in combat as a member of the Third Infantry Battalion, Stryker Brigade. However, according to newspaper reports about his background, Bales had an arrest record, specifically for a misdemeanor assault on a woman, a charge that was dropped after Bales agreed to undertake anger-management training. Whether the assault he committed pointed to resiliency issues or impulse control issues that would later feed into how he psychologically managed stress might very well come into play during his defense at his court martial. Bales was also involved in an automobile accident when he overturned his car. He blamed the accident on being overtired while driving and falling asleep at the wheel.

Bales was married to a woman he met online and had two children, a son and a daughter, and bought a house in Lake Tapps, Washington, near Joint Base Lewis-McChord. His expectation was that he would be promoted from staff sergeant to sergeant first class, which, in addition to raising his pay grade, might have kept him in the United States instead of putting him in line for another combat deployment. He was not promoted and was disappointed again when he was passed over for recruiting sergeant, a position that would have kept him close to his wife and family and enabled them to better manage their domestic situation and possibly their finances. Bales was seeking to avoid another deployment to combat, even though he had distinguished himself during three tours in Iraq.

Bales's disappointment at being rejected for promotion also had a direct impact on his financial situation. He did not get the monthly salary hike from going up another pay grade. The mortgage on his house in Lake Tapp was underwater because of declining property values, and he and his wife had put the house on the market to get out from under the financial burden. His finances were deteriorating rapidly, and now, after having been rejected for a promotion that would have kept him in Tacoma and improved his financial prospects, he was being redeployed to Afghanistan, leaving his wife alone to fend for the family while his house was in danger of foreclosure.

According to reports citing his lawyer as a source, Bales believed that his injuries—both his amputation and his brain trauma—should have reduced his medical fitness for duty to keep him in the United States. Bales's attorney told reporters that he doubted Bales would get a fair trial unless the entire prosecution is slowed down to the point where all evidence—including evidence that the two Afghans that prosecutors had listed as potential witnesses in the case turned out to be insurgents who were killed by U.S.-led forces, a claim that could not immediately be corroborated with U.S. military officials. Browne said he had government documentation showing that personnel at Lewis-McChord's Madigan Medical

Center had found his client to be suffering from both Post-Traumatic Stress Disorder and a traumatic brain injury. He said the diagnosis was made in early 2012 before Bales was sent to Afghanistan on a deployment that ended abruptly with the events for which he is charged. Defense lawyers previously have said Bales had suffered a possible concussion from a bomb blast during a prior tour of duty in Iraq."[10]

Despite all the evidence of Bales's problems prior to his final deployment, not only was he redeployed, but he was sent to one of the deadliest places in Afghanistan, an isolated firebase where his job was force protection for a Special Forces unit training Afghan soldiers—soldiers that the Army had to be wary of because many of them had been known to aim their guns on the Americans dispatched to train them. Inside the infantry combat personnel, this became known as "green versus blue," with the Afghan troops turning their fire on their supposed allies, the American troops. It was an untenable and unsustainable situation, especially in light of the scheduled withdrawal of American combat forces in just over two years. In many ways similar to Vietnam, this would be a planned retreat, with over-deployed American regulars and National Guardsmen needed at home fighting a rearguard action. And Bales was part of that rear guard, even as the Taliban ramped up to attack the withdrawing U.S. forces. Bales knew he was getting short, and he knew (as well as any soldier would at this stage of his career) that he was in terrible danger as a member of a rear guard.

If Bales was disconsolate at having been deployed to Afghanistan, his situation might have seemed even more hopeless given his assignment to Camp Belambay in Kandahar Province, where, although Taliban activity had diminished over the previous year, there were still pockets of resistance. At least one soldier who knew the firebase suggested that, given the level of surveillance at the base, it would have been

---

[10] Laura L. Myers | *Reuters—thu,* Jan 17, 2013

difficult for anyone to have simply walked off as Bales did. But Bales did suggest to his wife in a communication the day before he left the base that he had endured a "hard day" the day before. His lawyer said that Bales had witnessed a soldier's leg being blown off by a landmine. There was also talk that the two villages themselves were hiding Taliban fighters, but were off limits because they were considered friendly villages. However, two witnesses to the killing were killed later by NATO forces as enemy combatants. "Friendly villages?" All of this leads to speculation. Might the level of hostilities and the dangerous situation Bales found himself in have created a stress level that the already despairing sergeant could not deal with? Was his drinking and use of steroids contributing to either a severely impaired judgment or diminished capacity? Or was it far worse? Might Bales have actually sought suicide—in this case, suicide by the proxy of enemy fire—in order to get out of a hopeless life situation because—given the financial woes of his family, possible foreclosure and bankruptcy, anger at the Army for betraying him by denying him his promotion and the posting as a recruiting sergeant even after he completed training, and inability to fix his situation—he believed himself to be worth more dead than alive?

If he were actually contemplating suicide by proxy, he might have believed, this time under the influence of alcohol, that by entering a village believed to be harboring Taliban fighters and opening fire, he would have exposed himself to the enemy and been shot. When it didn't work the first time in the village south of Camp Belambay, he went to another village north of Camp Belambay, where he committed the same crimes, hoping for the same outcome: He would be killed by the enemy. Finally, still under the influence of alcohol and realizing that his plans for suicide did not work, he collapsed face-down in a nearby field (where he was spotted by surveillance cameras) until he regained his composure, got up, and returned to base, where he was taken into custody.

If suicide by proxy is a plausible explanation for Bales's seemingly inexplicable actions, what might his underlying mental condition have been, and might that condition be enough to form the basis of an insanity defense? The answers to this question lie in the definition of insanity as a criminal defense, the definition of insanity as it relates to fitness for duty, the insanity defense at court martial, and the standards of evidence for intent to commit suicide—or, at least, a symptom of Post-Traumatic Stress Disorder so severe that it obviates the mental intent, or mens rea, to commit a crime.

Any analysis of the crime and the motivation for that crime must start with an analysis of the psychiatric condition of Staff Sergeant Bales himself and the types of issues (including Post-Traumatic Stress Disorder and post-concussive brain trauma) that might have been affecting his decision-making process and his ability to distinguish reality from imagination on that morning of March 11, 2012, particularly if he was prescribed the antimalarial drugs. To address this issue, one must try to understand the overwhelming impact of combat trauma on the mind of a wounded warrior, who has no pre-service history for propensity to commit murder and mayhem on the scale just described—in fact, quite the opposite, from his combat history as reported. He tried to prevent collarteral damage to civilians.

Certainly, the prosecution can dig up prior charges against the defendant, especially those involving violence and substance or alcohol abuse. There was an apparent domestic violence assault prior to his marriage, as well as a history of substance abuse while stationed at Fort Lewis and even a hit-and-run incident. There was evidence of bad decisions in real estate and the experience of being one of the millions of Americans threatened with bankruptcy from overleveraging in the housing market. Very few would have suspected a precipitous drop in the Seattle/Tacoma metro market, one of the strongest economies in the world.

On the other hand, none of his commanders either at Fort Lewis or in Iraq noticed any propensity for such mass murder and mayhem throughout his combat career: three deployments in Iraq involving heavy near hand-to-hand combat, then readiness center preparedness for a fourth deployment (which was likely out of his zone of experience), and finally his duty in Afghanistan. Sure, it was a remote outpost, but he was not the highest-ranking soldier on base, nor was he the only American on base. Now the prosecution must find it necessary to discover the evidence of his being a bad soldier, and more, a mass murderer. Isn't that a bit like waking up one morning, like Liz Kendall, serial killer Ted Bundy's fiancée, to discover that you and your daughter had been cohabiting with one of this country's most notorious serial killers? That argument makes no sense. But, until Seargant Bales returned to his remote forward operating base and allegedly confessed to what he had done that night of March 11, 2012, nobody appeared to have noticed anything alarming about this soldier. Even neighbors in Tacoma said they were in shock over the reports of Bales's crimes.

His commanders also evidently had no doubts about his capabilities. Staff sergeants are the backbone of a fighting unit, providing support to their officers and bolstering morale of the troops. And to qualify as a sniper—a position that all but guarantees a close acquaintanceship with killing—he also underwent and passed routine psychological screening assessments. Bales's Army comrades have been quick to come to the support of the soldier they had known before Sunday. Capt Chris Alexander, his platoon leader in Iraq, said in an interview on Friday night that the sergeant "saved many a life" by never letting down his guard during patrols. "Bales is still, hands down, one of the best soldiers I ever worked with," he said. "There has to be very severe [post-traumatic stress disorder] involved in this. I just don't want him seen as some psychopath, because he is not."[11]

---

[11] By Philip Sherwell, New York, *The Telegraph*, March 17, 2012

Bales's wife, Karilyn Bales, broke her silence in an interview with NBC's Matt Lauer of the Today show. "It is unbelievable to me. I have no idea what happened, but he would not—he loves children. He would not do that," she said in excerpts released Sunday.[12]

Bales's actions were about to become so monstrous that the United States Cabinet most likely had to develop a contingency plan for leaving Central Asia before Force Protection of remaining troops from the President's surge became another nightmare like Dunkirk, the Battle of the Bulge, or more in our consciousness, the disastrous evacuation of our embassy in Saigon in 1975. One wonders, how could such a volcano erupt in the Army without any noticeable seismic shocks or steam emanating from a seasoned soldier assigned to one of the Army's most elite and battle-hardened brigade, The Stryker Brigade of Joint Base McChord-Fort Lewis and then for force protection of a remote and vulnerable Special Forces compound?

Absent all the facts of this case and Bales's life history, one must attempt to answer this question from an experience of having practiced psychiatry at Joint Base Lewis-McChord while Bales was decompressing with his Stryker Brigade and Special Forces Unit following the surge in Iraq in 2007. Sergeant Bales received most of his medical care for wounds received in three deployments at Madigan Army Medical Center in Tacoma, Washington. A practicing psychiatrist at Madigan would likely have examined Bales and his comrades from the Stryker Brigade returning from the surge in Iraq and would have had to familiarize himself or herself quite rapidly with the mission, risks, and threats to body and mind. A few of the men examined at Madigan were grossly psychotic, meaning that they were delusional. Being delusional, they were not able to discriminate external reality from internal voices, an

---

[12] Robert Bales Charged: Military Works To Limit Malaria Drug In Midst Of Afghanistan Massacre Posted: 03/25/2012 11:50 pm Updated: 04/ 5/2012

internal belief system that had taken them over, or auditory or visual hallucinations. One driver, call him Jedd, was actively talking with an imaginary friend, whom we can call "Dragon-man." The clinical psychologist who had been working with this unit for years said, "This man's psychotic. We need to medical board him out." Accordingly, proceedings for the Medical Evaluation Board were started immediately on Jedd.

So, what does this have to do with Bales, since nobody has ever said that he was psychotic? It has to do with what is known as Disintegration Anxiety, the worst imaginable emotional pain a person can experience. And it may directly impact the Bales case. What's Disintegration Anxiety like? Here's an example case study. It's a true story.

A patient named Ann came to her first appointment with Dr. Jones. She was impressed by the shiny floors and the modern, high-tech elevator bank of the brand-new medical office tower. No doubt she had selected a successful psychiatrist, and she felt fortunate to be able to see him. As the elevator silently and smoothly ascended, stopping a few times en route to her destination (the seventeenth floor), she started feeling a sense of tingling. Her heart began pounding against her chest. Ann was wondering if she would make it to her appointment without suffering unbearable physical reactions. She had an elevator phobia but expected to have that cured by Dr. Jones. She could overcome the rides, because of a hope for relief from her crippling anxiety, which neither she nor anyone else could comprehend. She led a pretty normal life, certainly no major traumas to cause anything like the severe anxiety attacks she was beginning to experience inside the tight confines of the slowly moving elevator.

The bell softly pinged at seventeen, and she stepped out onto the comforting thick carpeting, still fresh with the smell from just being unrolled. There was the welcoming sign on the glass waiting room door: "Dr. Edmond Jones, Psychiatrist."

She could see the door to his office open, and a young lady nodded good-bye to the receptionist, who obviously knew her well. This would be good, Ann thought, as she stepped into the waiting room, grasping the door opened by the last patient.

"Dr. Jones can see you right now," the receptionist said. She could tell that Ann was scared and tense.

Dr. Jones was finishing up writing in the last patient's chart and looked up briefly to nod his acceptance of Ann's entrance. Before he had a chance to introduce himself, Ann bolted for the window, wrenched it open, and threw herself out. Dr. Jones abruptly raced to the open window in a feeble attempt to catch her, but she had already crashed into the traffic below. He was sickened and in a state of shock. Hearing the sirens, he fumbled through his messages and found the referral note on Ann: "Ann Smith, thirty-five-year-old married mother of three, referred by Dr. Simpson, PCP, for panic attacks."

That would be the last patient Dr. Jones ever encountered in this building. The remainder of his career was at ground floor. Indeed, he knew patients with panic attacks could, and sometimes would, hurl themselves out the window as if they were flying without checking what's below, even when they were not suicidal. There was no medical or experiential evidence that Ann was or had been suicidal, or Dr. Jones would have taken special precautions.

Trained during the 1960s, Dr. Jones knew that very rarely, patients dropping LSD tabs became delusional in believing that they could fly like a bird. They had done the same thing Ann just did. In fact, stories abounded from college dormitories and residence halls, such as the Brittany Residence Hall at NYU in 1967, where students tripping on LSD tried to fly out of windows or off balconies because Jesus or an angel was beckoning them. But Dr. Jones consoled himself by thinking it was too rare in LSD abusers to expect any one of them to do it. Same thing with Ann. So, what was it about Ann's anxiety? Dr. Jones's whole career would be dominated by that question. It was a question that would follow him, as it did other psychiatrists, from their work in private practice into practice with combat military veterans who'd experienced traumatic events during the chaotic violence of combat.

These traumatic events can have the effect of splitting, or differentiating, parts of an individual's personality off from other parts of their personality, dissociating them and disintegrating the entire personality. As with Jedd, there can even be a serious psychosis in a person not otherwise predisposed to becoming psychotic. In other words, they are neither Schizophrenic nor Manic Depressive. They were simply overwhelmed with trauma that totally disintegrated their core "self."

The crush of violence can be what holds the fragile self together when threatened by Disintegration Anxiety. For example, Jedd was in heavy combat in Baqubah, Iraq during the surge. For those psychiatrists who had seen many soldiers from the battle for Baqubah, when they hear this name, they may flash back and see many of the faces of those soldiers who had fought there. One, "Whitey," along with another soldier who was his friend, was about to enter a house from which sniper fire was pinning down a Stryker Brigade unit. Suddenly the house exploded. Whitey's buddy, kicking open the door, tripped the wire of a booby trap, and this buddy's body parts came flying right into Whitey's face and past his ears. Whitey was splattered with blood, viscera, and organ parts. Other soldiers from the Stryker Brigade, who fought hand-to-hand with ferocious ragtag Sunni insurgents determined to fight to their death, also experienced bloody chaotic experiences.

The overwhelming firepower and mobility of the Stryker Brigade at Baqubah finally suppressed the insurgents' fire, but occupying and pacifying this city would be another matter. That is how General Petreus became famous—by co-opting the brutal Arab fighters, turning enemies into situational allies. Anyone who had spoken in depth to those soldiers from the Stryker Brigade fighting in Iraq can still imagine seeing the bloodbath that ensued during that battle. "The nastiest place on earth," as psychiatrists were known to describe Baqubah between appointments. Sometimes, they would share case histories with other therapists, just to clear their own minds before the next horrific combat history from the 2007 surge in Iraq.

Was Robert Bales in this battle? Was he ever in Baqubah? It is very possible he was. Units moved around very rapidly in country to back up units already on the ground and getting hit hard. Soldiers like Bales could have been in many different battles in many different regions of Iraq during what became known as "the surge." In fact, that mobility of units across country to back up other units was what the surge of reinforcements really was.

Our examplar soldier, Jedd, was there, and that is when "Dragon-man" saved him. At least that's what Jedd said; his clinical psychologist believed, as did his psychiatrist, that Jedd had been delusional during the battle of Baqubah. And another soldier, Whitey, was there, the soldier who watched when his buddy tripped the booby-trap bomb and was blown into body parts right into Whitey's face.

Whitey was so anxious every time the cannons fired on base that he literally fled from the parade ground during formation. Finally he was sent to a Madigan psychiatrist for a fitness for duty examination. There was a lot of tolerance for the warriors from the Stryker Brigade returning from the surge. There was even a warrior transition unit based in the hospital that helped them readjust. Still, they had to be at morning formation, and Whitey could not be standing in the open like that with cannons firing in the background, even though he knew they were ceremonial. But the small arms ratta-tat-tat from the nearby Special Forces compound was not ceremonial. It was the real thing.

Sergeant Bales was likely one of those soldiers doing training firing, too. And, when thinking of Jedd or Whitey—seeing Jedd tossed around in his Stryker from the blast of an IED, or that house exploding on Whitey and his buddy, who was ripped to pieces—

anyone who had treated these soldiers suffering from PTSD upon their return from Iraq would think of "Baqubah, the nastiest place on earth." It seared into the soldiers' psyches, penetrated their dreams, and affected neural pathways in their brains that would resonate and color reality well after the echoes from the guns had died away. But those echoes would still be in their minds.

There might have been many patriotic reasons for Robert Bales's enlistment after September 11th, reasons that overrode the financial services regulatory trouble that his company was in. There might also be a deeper issue. Perhaps some men are drawn to the unique beat and camaraderie of the combat world. Think of the altruism and patriotism evidenced by the young recruits in books or feature films such as *All Quiet on the Western Front, The Grand Illusion, Apocalypse Now, Platoon,* or *Full Metal Jacket,* an altruism quickly shattered by the brutal reality of war. Submerging one's individuality and privacy into the regimen of the military and then plunging into combat has something fundamental to do with one's identity. During periods of identity crisis, particularly before establishing careers, families, some measure of comfort in their own skins, or when those initial careers seem to fail, many find the warrior identity—or at least the atmosphere of excitement, danger, and heroic control over helplessness, particularly in wake of September 11th—alluring, and very likely, seductive. So did Bales. He enlisted and then honed his skills as an advanced infantry warrior, proving himself to be the man he needed to prove he was.

Back when he enlisted, however, he did not know about Whitey, and the absolute brutality of insurgent warriors in Iraq and Afghanistan. He had never heard of Baqubah and probably never imagined what would happen to Whitey and Jedd and the thousands of others who suffered the same fate. And certainly he would not expect to become so crazy that he would be depending on an imaginary friend like "Dragon-man" inside one of those modern killing machines called the Stryker. So, again, who really was Staff Sergeant Robert Bales?

What turned him into a monster of transcontinental proportions? Will his court martial ever reveal the full story? Probably not, because adversarial judge-determined courtroom justice has a way of covering up as much evidence as it reveals. Remember, even though a not guilty by reason of insanity verdict is almost unheard of under the Code of Military Justice, that verdict, if rendered, would almost immediately and irrevocably put every U.S. serviceman and woman in Afghanistan in mortal danger from the very troops of the Afghan National Army that they are trying to train.

We can understand the integrative power of war and violence, along with the disintegrative power of its unexpected horrors, by studying the works of psychiatrists Kohut and Chessick in threatened disintegration of the self. Some, like serial arsonist and clearly narcissistic Paul Keller in the serial arsons terrorizing Everett, Washington (just an hour-and-a-half up the road from Joint Base Lewis-McChord), disintegrate into murder and mayhem under an ordinary stress the rest of us simply take as life's expectable knocks.[13] The overwhelming majority of us, moderately well socialized and having overcome the psychological crises of our respective childhoods, develop the resiliency to deal with life's hard knocks without resorting to homicide or suicide. Others, like Paul Keller, suffer pathological narcissism. Humiliating bankruptcy was the straw that broke the camel's back in Keller's case, setting off the largest arson rampage in U.S. history.

Common stressors can therefore cause the disintegrative anxiety of a vulnerable narcissistic type like Paul Keller, who lit the state of Washington on fire just weeks from bankruptcy filing. And some are seriously mentally ill, like Virginia's Cho Seung-Hui in the massacre at Virginia Tech, Jared Loughner in the massacre at Safeway in Tucson (during which he shot and critically wounded Representative Gabrielle Giffords and murdered a federal judge

---

[13] Suicidal Mass Murderers: A Criminalogical Study of Why They Kill, CRC Press, 2011

and a young child), James Holmes in Colorado, white supremacist Wade Page in a suburb south of Milwaukee, and racist mass murderer Anders Breivik in the Norwegian massacre. Their last gasp for reintegration from their descent into the disintegrative anxiety of Schizophrenia is delusional consolidation. Schizpophrenia is something that, although horrific as it may seem to us, is better than the total annihilation anticipated in their total emotional collapse and then into explosions like super novas into psychosis and then into black holes of catatonic hallucinatory internal feedback loops, which is their final state.

For Staff Sergeant Robert Bales, however, and others committing atrocities in war, the act of integrating the disintegrating self through murder and mayhem becomes far more complex. Certainly it is rooted in childhood, genetic, developmental, and non-military stresses and challenges. But the necessary condition for such murder and mayhem is overwhelming combat trauma which, after being sought out as a solution, turns into an all-too familiar devil—and like Cho, Breivik, Loughner, and Page, explodes like a volcano.[14]

As much as people believe that trials bring out the truth, anyone who has practiced military law will tell you that often a court martial will cover up the truth because there are just too many secrets and hushed military issues to let them out into the open. In the case of Robert Bales (while armchair commentators may scream for his head), what may never be known is why this man was put back into the hot zone for yet another deployment, having suffered a traumatic brain injury and a foot amputation, been diagnosed with PTSD, and when in all likelihood, he was simply unfit for duty. No one is saying he didn't commit the crime. No one is saying a killer shouldn't face punishment. However, the Army should take an honest look at why he killed and what the red flags were that could have kept him from

---

[14] Pathological Narcissism, Suicidal Mass Murderers: A Criminological Study of Why They Kill, Liebert and Birnes, CRC, 2010

killing. And that's not asking too much of the military justice system. Technically—and deployment protocols must be highly technical—the base commander at Joint Base Lewis-McChord should have overridden his fitness for duty examination, which had to have such low numbers that it required such an override. Which brings up the ominous question: Was Robert Bales's fitness for duty profile updated prior to deployment to quantify his lower limb disability and neuropsychiatric disability? If not, there was a lapse in force health protection at this base that will require investigation. It is quite inconceivable that Seargant Robert Bales had a fitness for duty profile on his electronic health record that medically qualified him for the assignment for which he was deployed. It is simply inconceivable without direct intervention to override determination of unfit for deployment by the base commander. Thus, as a court martial jury prepares to send Robert Bales off to a firing squad, they might want to look at evidence that the Army, itself, and their own protocols are complicit in Bales's mental breakdown and likely attempt at suicide.

Chapter 5

Major Nidal Malik Hasan and Malignant Psychic Dissociation

After morning prayers at his local mosque near Fort Hood in Kileen, Texas, on November 5, 2009, shortly after 7:00 a.m., United States Army major and psychiatrist Nidal Malik Hasan said good-bye to some of his fellow worshippers. He asked for forgiveness from them, telling one person that he would not be back because he would be "traveling." That afternoon, at about 1:20, he entered the medical processing center at Fort Hood, the base where he was stationed. None of the personnel in that medical facility challenged Major Hasan's presence. He belonged there. He was a medical officer. Dr. Hasan was quiet at first, sitting down at a table as if observing or preparing to do his job of evaluating personnel heading overseas to fight in the Middle Eastern wars. Then, according to witnesses in the processing center that day, Major Hasan bowed his head as if in prayer, as if acknowledging an awesome presence, while he uttered "Allahu akbar." Drawing a weapon he had purchased months earlier from a local gun dealer, he opened fire on the defenseless assemblage of troops.

According to witnesses, Hasan seemed to choose his targets. Although at first some of the soldiers in the processing center might have thought this was a training exercise, when they saw others fall and saw the blood running across the floor, they knew it was for real. As Hasan moved his gun from target to target, he seemed to look directly into the faces of his victims, deliberately making eye contact and choosing those individuals who were in uniform. He moved around the room as soldiers ran for cover, some hiding under tables, others lying on the floor amongst the dead and wounded. Hasan was like a reaper, pointing his gun at those in uniform and sparing those in civilian clothes.

As he continued his shooting spree, bodies began piling up, some actually spread over the backs of chairs as they flew backward from the impact of the rounds. Hasan would stop shooting, reload, and then hunt down the victims he had already wounded. Each time the shooting stopped, Hasan tried to pick up his targets where he had left off, making sure, it seemed, to shoot those soldiers who looked like they might escape the carnage. In one case, Hasan saw a soldier try to cover another soldier who had been hit. Hasan walked over and poured three rounds into the soldier providing cover, wounding him critically.

At one point, chasing a soldier who had tried to escape outside the building, Hasan took aim again. And that was when the first police unit arrived. The car pulled up and Police Sergeant Kimberly Munley got out and immediately took after Hasan, firing as she went. They exchanged gunshots, wounding one another, but Hasan was critically wounded and fell to the ground. The carnage, lasting less than ten minutes, had ended.

Although he had begun his morning in peaceful prayer, Hasan was, by all accounts, an angry man, seething with uncontrollable fury about the U.S. role in the Middle East against his fellow Muslims. He had told relatives a year earlier that soldiers at bases where he was stationed had harassed him because he was a Muslim—he was of Palestinian descent—and now he feared he would be sent to Iraq or Afghanistan where, he believed, the Army was wantonly killing Muslims. Hasan was conflicted. Moreover, according to a statement from a family member, although he himself had not been deployed outside the United States, as a psychiatrist he had likely evaluated scores of soldiers returning from the Middle East and suffering from varying degrees of Post-Traumatic Stress Disorder—and he knew the terrifying horrors of the conflicts in Iraq and Afghanistan.

It was on that fateful November 5, 2009, that Dr. Hasan, possibly suffering from a complete personality breakdown and out of control, wearing his uniform and armed with an automatic pistol, opened fire on the soldiers waiting to be examined. Much like the mass murders who came before him—such as Cho Seung-Hui at Virginia Tech, or Wade Page in Milwaukee, stalking members of the local Sikh community—Hasan mercilessly mowed down almost 100 soldiers, killing thirteen and wounding eighty-six. Repeating "God is great" in Arabic, as if he were a martyr in the act of self-sacrifice, Hasan, possibly to his dismay, survived the gunshot wounds he received from the police, but was paralyzed from the waist down.

Was it overwhelming rage that drove him to commit these murders of soldiers being processed either for deployment to the Middle East or returning from their deployment? It's one thing to be resentful about orders that one believes must be followed. It's another thing to vent that wrath upon soldiers who have committed no crimes other than wearing the same uniform as their intended killer. Were there outside forces propelling the already sick mind of Dr. Hasan to commit a mass murder? Were there internal voices or auditory hallucinations roiling his anger and inciting him to violence? It is the latter that will determine at trial whether Dr. Hasan is deemed to be sane or insane. For capital punishment to be imposed on the killer, the prosecution must show that a defendant acted with rational premeditation and intent to commit the crime.

As a matter of law under the USCMJ, defendant Hasan is precluded from pleading guilty to a capital crime. Military law requires an automatic default plea of not guilty, placing the burden squarely upon the prosecution to prove beyond a reasonable doubt that the defendant formed the rational intent to commit the crimes charged and actually committed those crimes—mens rea and actus reus; a guilty mind and a guilty act. Thus, the defense will have to fall back on showing that there was either reasonable doubt that the defendant committed the crime—which is next to impossible because of the score or more of witnesses, including the wounded who saw him open fire—or that he was incapable of forming the mental intent to commit the crime by reason of insanity. And here is where the legal gears will mesh.

Dr. Nidal Hasan was of Palestinian descent, born in Alexandria, Virginia. His parents had emigrated from a town outside of Jerusalem and eventually relocated to Roanoke, Virginia, where they bought a restaurant and convenience store. An honors student at Virginia Tech, Hasan entered Army officer training school, graduated, received his commission, and was sent to Walter Reed Army Medical Center. He received his M.D. and completed his residency in psychiatry, all while being paid and receiving full benefits as an officer. He also received a master's degree in public health with a specialty in disaster psychiatry. By all accounts, Major Hasan, who moved through the ranks relatively quickly, should have been a well-trained officer, and particularly well prepared for his role as a psychiatrist dealing with the emotional and neurological stresses of troops returning from combat or in screening troops for combat. In addition, his Arabic and Muslim background made him a special asset to the military. But something went very wrong.

First, according to accounts that emerged after his arraignment, Nidal Hasan had enlisted in the Army against the wishes of his parents after graduating from Virginia Tech. They had opposed his decision to join the Army. It was 1995, and the United States was not only at peace with the rest of the world, but President Bill Clinton had formed a NATO coalition to protect the Muslim population in Bosnia after Serbian President Milosovich waged a war of "ethnic cleansing" against them. The United States Army did not itself have significant boots on the ground in the Serbian war, relying on air power to destroy the Serbian army. The first Gulf War against Iraq had also been waged a couple of years earlier under President George H. W. Bush (arguably with the full support of Arab countries, particularly Saudi Arabia) against Saddam Hussein's invasion of Kuwait. The United States was not at war with Islam, and in fact, had armed and supported the mujahadeen, or freedom fighters, in Afghanistan, helping them fight the Soviet invaders.

By 2003, however, when Dr. Hasan was completing his medical training, things had changed. After the attacks on September 11th, the U.S. had entered a ground war against both Afghanistan and Iraq. Hasan suddenly found himself as a medical officer in an Army waging war against Muslim governments, deploying missile-firing drones and using air strikes to hit targets, some of which resulted in civilian casualties, including women and children. Perhaps, Hasan thought, his parents were right. But whether they were or weren't, Hasan sought to get out of the Army, after the Army had poured hundreds of thousands of dollars into his military and medical training and likely had plans for using his unigue background as an asset. Hasan probably thought that it was impossible to get out of his contract with the Army, even though it was also possible that, with the correct legal arguments, he could have found a way. But the only way he could have been discharged early from his contract was from a medical retirement based on a psychiatric disorder. Such a way out of military commitment is extremely unpopular with the

Department of Defense. It would be even more scrutinized with a psychiatrist suspected of making up the symptoms for a lifetime of benefits as a retired military officer, and one whom they had trained, only to receive nothing back in the way of service. It is not certain whether he would have been allowed to collect disability payments to practice psychiatry in some venue in the civilian world. Service-connected veterans on full benefits are allowed to work at any job. But this would be different. It is possible that Dr. Hasan could have practiced in some way as a civilian psychiatrist while collecting benefits as a medically retired officer. One reason professionals stay in the military is to ultimately retire early with a good retirement and resume for their careers in civilian life. Dr. Hasan could have been perceived as scamming the system with an early retirement. However, Hasan knew everything about the technicalities of a medical evaluation board and likely considered medical retirement as an option, but the advice he sought told him it was not possible. As he looked at the hopeless situation he found himself in, his psychological condition deteriorated.

The question of intent might be resolved by Hasan's actions before the shooting rampage. For example, the prosecution might point out that Hasan purchased the weapon used in the shooting just a few days after he arrived at Fort Hood. He did not use a service weapon, but used $1,100 of his own money to purchase the murder weapon. Prosecutors might highlight Hasan's very outspoken opposition to the wars in the Middle East where he, even though not stationed there, was part of the machinery that sent soldiers there to fight Muslims. To those who knew him at the apartment complex where he lived, Hasan evidenced no hostility. He was neighborly and friendly, although to worshippers at his mosque, he was bitter and angry about his treatment in the Army: the harassment he claimed he faced because he was a Muslim, and his emotional conflict over helping to kill fellow Muslims by preparing and medically ministering to troops.

In the FBI report on the investigation into Hasan's crimes—a report headed up by Judge William Webster, former director of the FBI and director of intelligence at the CIA—Hasan's email communications with Sheikh Anwar al-Awlaki document and seem to show evidence of Hasan's gradual acceptance of suicide attacks. The emails were tracked by the FBI and Homeland Security, but the reviewers believed that Hasan, who was being transferred from Walter Reed to Fort Hood in 2009 for the purposes of preparing troops for deployment to Afghanistan, was simply researching Islamic law to prepare himself for giving advice to other Muslim soldiers.

In fact, the chair of psychiatry at Walter Reed, Dr. Hasan's boss, was of the opinion that Hasan's research on Islamic beliefs regarding military service during the global War on Terror "had extraordinary potential to inform national policy and military strategy." There were comments from his superiors that Hasan deserved promotion.

As Hasan's emails to al-Awlaki began to suggest that he would embrace suicide attacks if such attacks were in keeping with Sharia law, the authorities monitoring Hasan still did not believe he posed a threat. For example, on May 31, 2009, Hasan posted a message to al-Awlaki's website, saying:

"Assalum Alaikum Wa-RhamatuAllahi Wa-Barakatuhu brother Anwar; InshAllah Khair, I heard a speaker defending suicide bombings as permissible and have been using his logic in debates to see how effective it really is."

Also on May 31, 2009, Hasan sent a more extensive email to Al-Awaki, laying out specific details regarding his growing fascination with suicide attacks, trying to align them with the Koranic prohibitions against suicide. He maintained that speakers had told him that if suicide were an act of war against an attacker who was waging war against innocent victims, then suicide to stop those attacks or to engage in an eye-for-an-eye revenge was permissible.

"He contends that suicide is permissible in certain cases. He defines suicide as one who purposely takes his own life, but insists that the important issue is your intention. For example, he reported a recent incident where an American soldier jumped on a grenade that was thrown at a group of soldiers. In doing so, he saved seven soldiers, but killed himself. He consciously made a decision to kill himself, but his intention was to save his comrades, and indeed he was successful. So, he says this proves that suicide is permissible in this example, because the man is a hero. Then he compares this to a soldier who sneaks into an enemy camp during dinner and detonates his suicide vest to prevent an attack that is known to be planned the following day. The suicide bomber's [sic] intention is to kill numerous soldiers to prevent the attack in order to save his fellow people the following day. He is successful. His intention was to save his people and fellow soldiers, and the strategy was to sacrifice his life. The logic seems to make sense to me, because in the first example he proves that suicide is permissible (i.e., most would consider him a hero). I don't want to make this too long, but the issue of 'collateral damage,' where a decision is made to allow the killing of innocents for a valuable target. In the Qur'an, it states to fight your enemies as they fight you, but don't transgress. So, I would assume that suicide bomber whose aim is to kill enemy soldiers or their helpers, but also kill innocents in the process, is acceptable. Furthermore, if enemy soldiers are using other tactics that are unethical or unconscionable, then those same tactics may be used."

As his mental state deteriorated under the pressure of what he knew would be his deployment to a combat zone where he would be assisting in the fight against Muslims, it seems, from his emails to Al-Awlaki, that Hassan was attempting to use external rationalization to reinforce his internal suicidal ideations.

In psychiatry, this pathological defense is known as Projective Identification. It allows the projection of one's own homicidal rage onto another, thus justifying acts of lethal rage and even murder. It is a necessary defense for war to justify the dehumanization and killing of the enemy, but when it fails, a more deadly defense takes over, which is Identification With the Aggressor. This is what Nidal Hasan flipped to: the omnipotent and invincible al-Qaeda jihadist killing about as many American soldiers as any jihadist ever had. Did he guarantee himself a seat beside his comrades hijacking airplanes to destroy the United States government en route to an eroticized paradise with myriad virgins? We may never get the answer to this question, because Major Hasan actually failed in his jihadist mission. He is alive, paralyzed, and possibly looking at a long life deep in the bowels of a very unfriendly Fort Leavenworth Prison, unless the Army decides to execute him.

At seeming odds with the violence that Hasan perpetrated at Fort Hood was a story told by one of his relatives to the *New York Times* about Hasan's caring for a small bird he had adopted. He allowed the bird to eat partially chewed food off his tongue. When the bird died, Hasan buried the bird and went into mourning for months. Was this the same person who imagined himself as a suicidal martyr as the only way out of performing his duty in Afghanistan? Perhaps, defense may argue, Hasan was suffering from a Dissociative Disorder brought on by Identity Diffusion as he fought internally over the conflict between serving his country's armed forces and fighting against his own religious compatriots.

Hasan attempted to resolve his conflict by getting out of his military obligation, but was told by those who advised him that only the Secretary of Defense, Donald Rumsfeld, could get him out of his commitment. The Army needed medical personnel, he was told, especially officers of Arab descent, and because his commitment as a medical officer was seven years, given the amount of professional training the Army had provided, Hasan's chances of getting out of the Army were slim to none. Hasan reportedly told his cousin that he had accepted his fate and resolved to stay in the Army, although he was frustrated and angry about the direction things had gone.

Between 1998 and 2001, both of Nidal Hasan's parents died. Seeking peace after his losses, Hasan increasingly turned to religion.

His uncle remarked that Hasan had taken these losses with great difficulty and had become isolated from any social life. In his isolation, he found comfort in Islam and became increasingly devout. Perhaps this was where his turning against the Army began, especially in light of September 11th and the generally popular anti-Muslim reaction to it. In his loneliness, Hasan told those he knew at his mosque in the Washington area that he was looking for a wife—a woman, like him, of Arab descent. Although he asked the imams of his mosque for help, he found no one.

At-risk individuals, those in serious conflict—moral or otherwise—with themselves, and those coping with losses of loved ones are especially vulnerable to outside influences that speak to their losses. It is as if the loss and conflict create a black pit within the at-risk person's mind into which any seemingly solace-giving voice can take root. This is the reason why people in pain seek counseling from those they trust, either psychological counseling or religious counseling. This may explain Major Hasan's acute psychological vulnerability after the loss of his parents, his isolation, his failure to find a wife, and his growing moral conflict over the wars in Afghanistan and Iraq.

Hasan sought counseling from his mosque in Virginia, the imam of which was later designated as a terrorist: Anwar Al-Awlaki, a fiery speaker who incited his followers to oppose American operations in the Middle East, and who was killed in a CIA drone strike in Yemen in September 2011. This was an American war against Islam prosecuted by crusaders and Zionists, the imam said, a war that all righteous Muslims must oppose by any means necessary. American-born Al-Awlaki preached violent jihad against the United States, inciting not only Hasan, with whom he exchanged emails before the Fort Hood shooting, but also the now-infamous 2009 underwear bomber Umar Farouk Abdulmutallab and the 2010 Times Square bomber Faisal Shahzad, a Pakistani immigrant, both of whom pointed to Al-Awlaki as their sources of inspiration to violence. Although religious content speech in America is generally protected under the First Amendment, incitement speech is not, particularly incitement to commit violence. Al-Awlaki's incitement to jihad, a religious holy war in which all Muslims are ordered to fight against the United States, was not deemed protected speech, especially after acts of mass homicidal violence and attempted mass homicide were linked directly to the imam. Al-Awlak had declared himself an enemy combatant against the United States in a time of war.

Adding to Hasan's growing belief that he had to oppose the wars in Afghanistan and Iraq were his experiences in interviewing soldiers returning from the fronts. What he learned from those soldiers further deepened his beliefs. In fact, in a presentation he gave at a master's seminar on public health, Hasan explained why the War on Terror was, in actuality, a war on Islam itself. And it was Hasan's belief that a war on Islam was a war he had to oppose. Hasan became a proselytizer, arguing with anyone who would listen that the wars in the Middle East were wrong and had to be opposed.

Although Hasan's vehemence might have upset his classmates in the graduate program—upset them to the point of making complaints about him—none of them saw him as a terrorist or as a threat. At least that is what has been reported by the Pentagon. Rather, it was reported that he simply, according to his classmates, didn't look the type. But Hasan did have difficulties during his training at Walter Reed; difficulties that required some counseling. However, according to his supervisor there, nothing Hasan said indicated that he was intending to violate his oath of loyalty to the military. And, as records show, other medical personnel at Walter Reed sought and received counseling, indicating that counseling itself might have been considered routine at a high-stress medical facility. Moreover, other residents at Walter Reed said there were other military doctors there who had expressed opposition to the war. Yet no expressions of opposition sounded anything like those of Dr. Hasan!

After his posting to Fort Hood from Walter Reed, a base from where soldiers would be routinely sent to Afghanistan or Iraq, Dr. Hasan, now a newly-appointed major, realized that he might be in line for deployment in the Middle East. In fact, he may have known that he was going to be deployed as a means to simply get him to a place where his troubles could be handled in less administratively complex manner. It could even have been more insidious, because his opposition to the war once he was in Afghanistan would have put him at odds not only with his command, but also with enlisted personnel, and might have gotten him "fragged."

He found an apartment near the base and bought himself an automatic handgun at a local gun dealership, according to federal law enforcement records. Hasan generally kept to himself in his new apartment, which is not to say he was in the least bit hostile to anyone. His neighbors remarked that he was friendly, always greeting people and being respectful to them, and once offering a ride to a neighbor who needed it. And although he had a bumper sticker on his car that read "Allah is Love," which prompted a newly repatriated soldier to run a key along the length of Hasan's car, Major Hasan did not file a formal complaint with the police. He seemed almost unfazed by it, as if the harassment he endured earlier in his military career had inured him to the insult. As the possibility of deployment to Afghanistan loomed larger in his mind, he had bigger worries to deal with, particularly being attacked by his own troops, which was not uncommon in Vietnam.

At Fort Hood, Dr. Hasan came face-to-face with the very soldiers who were being deployed to fight and kill enemy fighters in Iraq and Afghanistan. He likely did fitness for duty exams on soldiers returning, thus hearing their traumatic experiences and even bitterness towards other Muslims. And on the inpatient unit, he saw the sickest of the returning soldiers. These were likely his two main duties as a psychiatrist at Fort Hood. He probably did not do extensive psychotherapy of PTSD patients, because that procedure is usually in the realm of psychologists and social workers trained in psychotherapy. Psychiatrists were needed for emergency psychiatry, inpatient psychiatry and forensic psychiatry—the latter of which was to determine whether a soldier should be disciplined for a violation or complaint from his commander, or medically discharged from the military with a pension worth millions in lifetime benefits.

In Hasan's swelling belief system, these troops were killing Muslims who were fighting in their own homelands against invaders. His job at the Fort Hood medical center was to assess the psychological fitness for duty of soldiers being deployed and diagnosing the more serious cases returning from war, enabling, in his mind, the very invasion and killing he was vigorously opposed to, because every effort was encouraged for psychiatrists to return soldiers to duty. As he performed this job, in his mind, he was sending soldiers to the front to kill Muslims—but he also prayed five times a day at a nearby mosque. He was a man clearly caught in conflicting roles: a devoutly loyal practicing Muslim, and a military officer who'd sworn a loyalty oath to his native country, its army, and his own medical profession.

As he wrestled with his conscience, seeking a way through the morass of opposing loyalties, he asked the founder of the mosque he attended—a retired Army sergeant who had seen combat in the Gulf—how he should resolve his conflict and counsel Muslim soldiers going to Afghanistan and Iraq who might be struggling with the same issues plaguing Dr. Hasan. The sergeant, Osman Danquah, explained that this was a volunteer army. Nobody forced these soldiers, nor did anyone force Hasan, to join. Once they joined, they had to follow orders unless they sought to declare themselves conscientious objectors—a way out that many young men sought during the Vietnam War draft years. It would have been way too late for that in Hasan's case.

Ultimately, Hasan decided that he would not go to Afghanistan, no matter what the cost. He said that because the Koran stated that if a Muslim fought and was killed in the military against other Muslims, especially if he were fighting alongside Christians and Jews, he would go to hell. Thus, Hasan's mind was made up. He would not go to the Middle East. On the night before the shooting, he had mustered his resolve. He would be a martyr and commit jihad.

How to represent that martyrdom in court is the issue facing defense counsel, because ultimately Dr. Hasan did not achieve his goal of suicide. What are the explanations, the diagnoses, and the legal defense? First, was Hasan suffering from PTSD? He had not been in combat, not been deployed to the Middle East, and had spent the majority of his career in the Army in officer and then medical training. He spoke to soldiers who had been in the Gulf, but had no firsthand experience there. However, if he was not suffering from PTSD, the fear of going to a place where his serving in an Army fighting Muslims was a capital sin might have predisposed him to severe stress born out of that fear. And he likely knew that he had a good chance of killing and being killed, possibly by his own troops. Thus, it was more likely that he was suffering from what psychiatrists call "Identity Diffusion," more technically known as Dissociative Disorder NOS.

Hasan may have even been one of the rare cases of Multiple Personality Disorder as he tried to cope with two violently opposed conflicting loyalties: two warriors who, in the case of Multiple Personality Disorder, did not even know of the existence of the other. Certainly Hasan's observing ego had strong revolutionary roots from inside his family culture. The Palestinians, exploited by other Arab countries, co-opted by the ruling Hashemite Jordanians, and thus living as an occupied people, were stateless. Technically, after World War II, Palestine didn't even exist as a national territory. It was called "Transjordan," but would have become Palestine after the 1947 UN resolution partitioning the British Palestine mandate, had not the Arab states rejected the mandate and started a war. Thus, the country of Palestine, brought into existence as a modern Arab and Islamic state by UN Resolution 181, never came to be. Instead, the Palestinians became refugees on what should have been their own land.

Accordingly, for Nidal Hasan, military training and impending combat duty might have been like creating a fight to the death behind two warrior states of mind: one, the Palestinian anti-Zionist warrior, and the other, the counter-terrorist warrior, which for our purposes could be considered the hypnotic trance of military preparedness for robotic destructiveness. Could Hasan's observing ego, the anti-Zionist revolutionary, have selected the Fort Hood preparedness center by coincidence, or did he find himself there, much to his chagrin, as the launch point for his own crucible of fighting Muslims in a Muslim country?

Although he was a first-generation Palestinian-American, Hasan, by his own admission, had an observing ego buried in his mind that prohibited warring with Muslims. This is what he told friends at his mosque, as well as his imam. As a psychiatrist, he would have been aware of his own internal conflict from the perspective of an outsider, even as he tried to grapple with it internally. It was like listening to a voice while observing clinically that there was a voice. Add to this morass the real external voice of the violently anti-American Al-Awlaki abjuring him from contributing to and suborning any violence against Muslims. In Hasan's mind this was irreconcilable. There could be no finessing this problem.

There is no doubt that Al-Awlaki did the psychic driving to activate Hasan's observing, or alter, ego. Much like a multiple personality, Hasan was splitting into two conflicting warriors. He was a Muslim doctor inculcated with opposing oaths: He had taken the Hippocratic Oath to do no harm while also counseling soldiers to do harm to the very people who wanted to harm Americans. These ego states, with Al-Awlaki's skilled enabling, were actively pitted against each other in such a way that no matter where Hasan turned for counseling, it offered no resolution. He was trapped in ever-hardening psychological aspic.

Certainly all the psychiatrists working with him had to have known he was coming apart. Given Hasan's disintegration, the Army command, knowing that Hasan was actively looking for a way out and causing a disturbance in the otherwise smooth chain of command, did what they sometimes do in the army—sunsetted him to Fort Hood, probably assuming his deployment, as in case of Staff Sergeant Robert Bales, would take care of matters once and for all with a sink-or-swim resolution.

Sometimes, especially in legal cases, unexpected things come out in the wash. So it may come to be regarding the psychological issues surrounding Hasan and how they apply to all pending litigation, civil as well as criminal. For example, while the Army assembles its criminal case against Dr. Hasan, the survivors are suing the Army. At issue in a civil case, was the Army itself negligent in breaching its duty of care to troops being deployed overseas by allowing a mass murderer into the processing unit? Did the Army, because of Hasan's open dissatisfaction with his status in the Army and the Army mission in the Middle East, have what can be construed as legal notice of an impending danger to those troops harmed in Hasan's assault? Could the assault be construed as workplace violence, where other workers have successfully sued the proprietors of the workplace for not providing adequate protection? Or will the government argue that military personnel, by the very nature of their volunteering for service, give an implied consent to be confronted by danger no matter where it occurrs? And does said consent thereby absolve the government of any liability in a wrongful death or other type of negligence suit?

If the suit is not dismissed, maybe there is some information about Hasan in plaintiff's hands already, even as the Army assembles its case against Hasan and Hasan's attorneys prepare their insanity defense, all of which will play in the victims' suit against the Army. Compounding the legal problem is the recent declaration of President Obama that the Fort Hood shooting was indeed workplace violence, and not specifically a military matter of soldiers always having to expect being in harm's way.

The Dissociative Disorder Defense and How it Relates to Nidal Hasan and Robert Bales

The question in Multiple Personality Disorder (MPD) cases—and also in any cases based on committing felony violence in a dissociated state that is not the true persona of the defendant—is pretty clear: "Who am 'I'?" Worse, who is the "I" around whom a case revolves?

For example, one evening after work, Joe might be the grouchy guy at a corner table hunkering over a beer. He may be the guy who looks at every woman in the bar, but gets angry because he can't figure out what to say to them—whether he should sidle up to buy one of them a drink, sit silently and muse about the women he sees while stewing in his own frustration, or simply cast nasty glances around the bar, avoiding eye contact with someone bigger than he is, until he decides to go home. You might not even notice him. But this is certainly not the same guy who goes to work in the morning, plunks down his change for a cup of coffee at the local 7-11, and then arrives at the office to deal with the vicissitudes of his job every day. Maybe he's the guy who, on weekends, watches football games on TV for ten hours each day and pays no attention to anyone else. He's no fun to be with. He's worse than a bore. He's an angry bore. Yet you might see him at a gas pump, at a doughnut shop at lunchtime, or even on the 7:26 from Princeton Junction to Penn Station and find him to be perfectly charming.

Who is Joe? Who is his "I"? Within the range of normality, Joe's personality differences may depend on when he slept, how much sleep he got the night before, and how well his day is going. But, in the normal world, Joe can remember being these different ego states of mind, and if one reminds him of when he was grouchy, when he was friendly, or when he simply zoned out with beer and chips in front of the Broncos game, he would remember. These are Joe's states of mind, or in psychiatric terms, his ego states. Joe is all of these personalities throughout the day—full of optimism in the morning, worn out by three after a late lunch, and simply grouchy and hostile to the world while standing on the platform waiting for the 5:56 train back home. Think of that same Joe personality on the 405 south into Orange County, California, fuming at the SUV just ahead of him with a lone driver and no passengers that slides into the special HOV lane and zips away. You'd wonder whether he'll take it out on his kids when he gets home. That's Joe, a guy of many minds and moods through the day—but an individual who can remember them, navigate among them, feel remorse, and even apologize if he's offended you. He can control them, because he's the only captain in the wheelhouse of his head.

However, what about the person who cannot recall any of these states of mind when he's engrossed in watching the football game? What if the grouchy guy, the guy in the office cubicle, the guy on the 405 or on the 5:56, and the guy dropping his pocket change into the charity dish at his church doesn't know, can't remember, and has no cognizance of any of the other personalities, and might be shocked if you were to bring up the differences? The patient to whom psychiatrists ask, "Do you lose time, as if you can't remember your birthday party last week or the camping trip over the weekend?" A "yes" to that question is a red flag for the patient who dissociates and may in fact have multiple personalities, or at least, as in combat veterans, a dissociated warrior state, ready for combat at any time when the environmental cues call him to action, even decades later. The warrior is still in there, but rarely visible to either an intimate or the veteran himself.

Consider, for example, a patient named Marcy, who was committed to the psychiatric service at a county hospital because she broke into the home across the street when hearing a child screaming in the middle of the night. When she first met her psychiatrist, she was polite, almost mild, cooperative, and not in the least bit emotionally intimidating. Marcy was physically quite striking—a tall and somewhat muscular black woman of whom one might become fearful, especially if she were breaking down your door.

Marcy related a coherent story about how she knew that child abuse was going on across the street from her. She said she could tell what was happening in her neighbor's house from the child's screams that carried across the street. The screams were all too familiar, because she remembered similar experiences in her own home when she was a child. Her father, she said, was a violent man when intoxicated, which was every weekend. She recalled getting all her little sisters together when she heard him coming home and hiding with them under the kitchen table. Sometimes her father would just fall on the couch and go to sleep. But sometimes he would take his drunken rage out on his children, especially Marcy, the eldest, the target child. In the parlance of family psychology in the late twentieth century, at the very least, Marcy was an ACOA, an adult child of an alcoholic. But, as her doctors would soon discover, that was not the worst of it.

It was her attending psychiatrist's responsibility to determine whether Marcy was dangerous to herself or others, the legal standard for commitment to a hospital's psychiatric facility. Her attending psychiatrist would be paged later in the day to testify in the county hospital superior courtroom about her mental condition and risk of imminent dangerousness to herself or others. While working up other admissions, her psychiatrist went to another ward in the hospital to see another new patient before returning to check on Marcy. Just then another psychiatrist pushed open the door while holding his head in pain.

"Damn, this woman is a criminal."

Marcy had ripped his clipboard from him and smashed him in the head with it, causing a severe bruise. At this point, with two psychiatrists having visited Marcy, there were two entirely different opinions about her safety: She was mild, and she was violent. After being called out on yet another emergency, her attending psychiatrist, the first to have interviewed her, soon received a page from Marcy's nurse.

"Doc, you need to get here right away. We have her in seclusion, but it's taking all the staff we have just to keep her from hurting one of us. And, Doc, ah . . ." There was a long and pregnant pause. "Marcy sounds like a man."

Marcy's attending psychiatrist rushed to the ward where he saw hospital staff workers trying to restrain this suddenly powerful woman. They had to be meticulously careful because security had recently restrained a patient who later died from asphyxia during their restraint procedures. Accordingly, security personnel were prohibited from coming onto the unit except for a near-riot. But there they were in a struggle with Marcy, just two hours after her psychiatrist had softly spoken with her, and just one half-hour after she had ripped the clipboard from another psychiatrist's hands. Marcy's face was ferocious, contorted in rage. Her eyes reddened as if inflamed.

"You better get the hell out of here, you goddamned motherfucker," she yelled at the psychiatrist in a deep baritone voice that was not at all contrived or affected. This was real, not an act. Her psychiatrist was staring into the face of what the victims had seen the night before.

Her attending psychiatrist administered emergency medication that sedated her, and by noon she was back out on the ward, quietly eating lunch with other patients. The doctors and psychiatric nurses held a conference on her behavior, and another psychiatrist—an elderly and somewhat frail-looking man with a black beret and strong European accent—offered to see her. Her attending psychiatrist watched as the elderly physician approached her, and she invited him to sit down. The staff personnel were all amazed that the elderly doctor and now-calm patient talked quietly through the lunch. And then the older psychiatrist came back to the nursing station.

"Did you get anything from her?" Her attending psychiatrist asked. The other psychiatrist who'd been hit with his clipboard was still pretty angry and insistent on calling the police and filing criminal charges.

"I did. She told me just what she told you," he said. "She went into the house to protect the child."

"What was the male voice and looks that could kill?" Her attending psychiatrist asked.

"She did not recall any of that, but noticed the marks on her arms from the struggle to restrain her."

The patient's inability to remember her behavior—as if some other person did it without her knowledge—sounded like Multiple Personality Disorder. But Multiple Personality Disorder was talked about more as fiction then as a reality by most doctors. Accordingly, her attending psychiatrist was a skeptic, as were many other psychiatrists, of the diagnosis of Multiple Personality Disorder popularized by the University of Kentucky College of Medicine in the story of Three Faces of Eve, a popular book in the 1950s and a motion picture starring Joanne Woodward as Eve White and Eve Black, with Lee J. Cobb as her psychiatrist. Multiple Personality Disorder had become a very popular legal defense during the 1960s, as well as the subject of many a television show. However, her psychiatrist had just read a study from Switzerland that strongly confirmed its existence as a mental illness.

In a survey of Swiss psychiatrists who were sent a list of criteria for the diagnosis of Multiple Personality Disorder, 90 percent responded. That was a robust number, and more significantly, the rarity of the disorder was confirmed. The statistical analysis predicted that the average psychiatrist would see at least one Multiple Personality Disorder patient in his or her career. Therefore, Marcy's psychiatrist knew that to see the switch—particularly the sudden, out-of-nowhere emergence of a male ego state in a seemingly normal woman—was gut-wrenching. And it was. Nobody can fake such a radical switch from one personality state to another. What the hospital staff had witnessed was the male alter ego of Marcy.

Marcy did not know that this male existed in her. It may have had a name, but no one picked up on that in all the excitement of the moment. It was perfectly clear to all, however, that this male alter ego was much stronger than the person named Marcy, who was interviewed earlier during her meeting session with the attending psychiatrist. And, indeed, research on true alter egos that have emerged from unmistakable switching have different physical capabilities. Their muscular tension is actually specific to each. What the individual alter egos know is different, and what they are told is remembered differently, often as a result of their state of mind—or ego state—when they learn the information. The research also shows a family history of altered states like Marcy demonstrated, as well as documented histories of Post-Traumatic Stress Disorder, most commonly from abuse when it can be detected. So, in the extreme and rare case of Marcy, we know she had at least two, if not three, compartmentalized personalities that were likely fairly complete identities. And they were compartmentalized to the point that they did not know each other. They were, in fact, dissociated from each other.

During Marcy's violent outburst, the staff may have also seen a third ego state that was a violent female. Marcy did not remember that third ego state either, although she could not dispute hitting one psychiatrist over the head with his clipboard and threatening bodily harm to her attending psychiatrist. The Jack—or Jacks—was back in the box after she had been sedated, and by the time she had spoken with the elderly psychiatrist, who, apparently, was a non-threatening figure to her. His interview with her calmed her down to the point that he was able to get a lot of history that none of the other staff could get from her; history medically relevant to the dissociation of her personality.

Of course, between the states of mind described here in "who I am" and Marcy, there is a broad spectrum of ego states that may fade in and out with little recollection of what happened. The Dissociative Experiences Scale is a self-administered questionnaire that, along with the Minnesota Multiphasic Personality Index, picks up lying and deception and has been very accurate in culling out the real dissociative patients from controls who play the role of dissociating after watching Three Faces of Eve. Likewise, tests of memory, brain wave tests, muscle tension testing, visual acuity, and even lazy eye separate the roleplayers from the dissociating patient, particularly an extreme dissociating patient like Marcy.

One wonders, therefore—as in the case of Robert Bales, who says he cannot remember the murderous events of March 2012—if it is possible that Dr. Hasan did not recall the shootings at Fort Hood until he himself was shot and found that he was unable to move? Are we talking about multiple personality events under the crushing stress of ego-destroying conflict? But how could this happen so far into a doctor's career in the military? There has been no report of child abuse in his background. He was never in combat. But we do know that Post-Traumatic Stress Disorder is intergenerational in transmission—in other words, it might not be generated only by situational stress, but by transmission from the experiences of a prior generation. In this case, it might have been transmitted by the experiences of Major Hasan's stateless parents.

Dr. Hasan was born in the United States, but his parents were Palestinian and most likely exposed to violence and hardship in the small West Bank villages, as well as the ongoing violence of war, Palestinian terror groups, and the Israeli Defense Forces reaction. Violence was, and is, an ongoing story on the West Bank, as well as in Gaza. It is possible that Dr. Hasan had what is known as an "observing ego" buried in him from his family background, and that "observing ego"—his alter—was causing a war inside him. Could he take going to war against Muslims?

Major Hasan's observing ego was very receptive to the preaching and incitement speech of Imam Al-Awlaki, and it grew and grew in his mind with every communication back and forth between his residency training program at Walter Reed Hospital and Yemen.

The alter ego was created, likely without Hasan's awareness, just by listening to or absorbing the experiences of his Palestinian family, and then grew like a malignant tumor in his mind until it became a closet jihadist. All of this for now is pure conjecture, but it explains what, until now, has only been called by military psychiatric experts an "anomalous suicidal mass murderer." It might not have been anomalous at all.

In the same way that Marcy's attending psychiatrist missed the dangerous male alter ego in Marcy when he first saw her—and even after she assaulted his colleague—the Army psychiatric colleagues and faculty missed the jihadist suicidal mass murderer threatening to take over the self of Major Nidal Hasan, psychiatrist in the United States Army. Perhaps he knew he was coming apart, just like the suicide-bent Staff Sergeant Bales might have. Both resisted deployment to Afghanistan. But, like Marcy, the rumblings of suicidal mass murderers in the psyches of both soldiers could not be heard.

History has recorded the rest, just as history will be archived in the court martial records: Two disasters of murder and mayhem from men not expected to explode in volcanic eruptions, as they did, but simply to go away, far away. They were to go away to one of the most turbulent, failed nation-states in the world, a remote piece of real estate that chewed up foreign armies from Alexander the Great and Genghis Kahn to the British Empire and the Soviet Union. It was a battlefield of feuding clans and Pashtun tribal alliances that few Americans could care less about—except that it was believed to be the location of Bin Laden's hiding place, in some of the most foreboding mountains and harsh terrain on earth, inhabited by war lords, drug dealers, and incomprehensible religious fanatics from another era. To go there in a U.S. Army uniform, you better have your head screwed on right. We know that neither Hasan nor Bales did.

Thus, will their defenses be dissociation? Will we learn what happened to cause seemingly good-enough career U.S. soldiers to go berserk? It is in the American public's interest to try to get all the facts that can be obtained. We know the prosecution will not be generous in allowing anyone to have them. That is the nature of the beast. Two atrocities committed by career soldiers cleared for deployment against such soft targets: helpless families sleeping in Afghan villages, and Hasan's own unarmed soldiers, a few of whom would be his patients, in the readiness center of Fort Hood. And, very likely, two career soldiers who were both victims of voices speaking inside their heads until—no matter how hard they tried to resist—they exploded in violent gunfire heard all around the world.

Chapter 6

The Strange Case of Dr. Timothy V. Jorden Jr.

What was it that lured Jacqueline Wisniewski into a basement stairwell corridor at the Erie County Medical Center in Buffalo, New York, on June 14, 2012? What did trauma surgeon Dr. Timothy Jorden, Wisniewski's ex-lover, say to her that convinced her to be alone with him? Perhaps we will never find out the nature of their last conversation. What we do know, however, is that once in the stairwell, the two of them all alone, Dr. Timothy Jorden fired five rounds from one of the weapons he had brought with him to the hospital directly into his ex-girlfriend's head, killing her instantly. He fled from the grounds of the medical center back to his Hamburg home in an affluent enclave on the shores of Lake Erie, then slid out the back door of his house into an area of dense underbrush less than a mile from his home and near the shore of the lake, where, now completely alone with whatever remorse and fury he felt, he put his .357 Magnum to his head and fired another round, ending his own life.

Police would discover his body after they had put out an alert across the country for this former Army Special Forces combat soldier who, they publicly warned, was armed and presumed very dangerous. Within two days of the manhunt for Jorden, police followed up on leads from a surveillance video that showed Jorden entering his home thirty minutes after Wisniewski's murder, then exiting from the rear of his home into the dense bushes. Following Jorden's path—having to rappel some of the way, due to steepness of the terrain—police discovered a body. It was Dr. Timothy Jorden. Case closed? Not at all. The manhunt may have ended with the discovery of Jorden's body, but the mystery of the crime still lingers.

According to law enforcement officials, the Buffalo police investigating the Wisniewski murder asked local Hamburg police to stake out Jorden's Hamburg home soon after determining that Jorden was a "person of interest" wanted for questioning in connection with the fatal shooting at the hospital. The officials said that Jorden was captured on surveillance cameras entering his home within an hour after the shooting. Then they lost track of him but believed he might have fled the area, which is why they posted a bulletin to other police forces to be on the lookout for him and warned his ex-wife in Lakewood, Washington. Apparently they believed that she, like his murdered ex-lover, had reason to fear for her life as well.

Initially police thought they had captured Jorden on surveillance video leaving the front of his Hamburg lakefront home, this time with a gun. However, police were in for another shock when it turned out that the man leaving the home wasn't Jorden after all. It was his old high school buddy, Buffalo police detective Martin Motley III, leaving the home wearing a yellow t-shirt and tan shorts. According to the *Buffalo News*, "When Hamburg police went to stake out the Lake View home of Dr. Timothy V. Jorden Jr., on Wednesday morning, they encountered an off-duty Buffalo cop coming out of the home." Motley was carrying a Rolex watch, a personal gun, and $5,000 in cash. According to police, Motley (who had been on injured sick leave for three years due to an on-duty injury) was taken into custody, brought back to the Buffalo police, and questioned about why he was at the house right after the murder, and of course, whether he knew the whereabouts of Timothy Jorden.

Motley's attorney, Roland Cercone, gave a statement to the press in which he explained that Martin Motley's only interest in going to the Jorden home after the shooting was that he was worried about his friend, Jorden, because the doctor was acting strangely, especially with respect to the multitude of gifts that he had purchased and was giving out to his friends. Why was he doing that? Motley said that he went to Jorden's home to find out why. He said that he had became concerned, and that was the reason he went to his friend's house. The attorney said that Motley was cooperating fully with the police, although the police released a statement in which they said that Motley was "not saying much" about why he was in the house, what prompted him to go there, or why he had the items, according to an article in the *Buffalo News*.

"We're trying to figure out why Motley was in the doctor's house. We know they have been good friends since their days at Bennett High School," one police official said.

Martin Motley III, 47, joined the city police force in 1988, according to city records. Before he went off on sick leave, Motley did patrol duty on the city's East Side and was also a member of the department's elite SWAT team, fellow officers said.

Police theorized that Dr. Jorden, who friends and neighbors said seemed to have declined physically over the last few months, had become so distraught over his breakup with Jackie Wisniewski that he killed her. He had lost weight, one neighbor said, and the difference was obvious. It was as though Jorden had gone into a "tailspin" since his breakup with his girlfriend, one neighbor told the *Buffalo News*.

While workers at Erie County Medical Center mourned both Jackie Wisniewski and her killer, Timothy Jorden, they were left with what seemed, to many of them, a paradox. On the one hand, Dr. Jorden was well-respected as a trauma surgeon, having saved, according to one hospital employee, "thousands of lives." Others described him as a dedicated surgeon who was loved by his patients. His friends couldn't reconcile Jorden's murdering his girlfriend and his own suicide. Was it only his breakup that prompted him to commit the murder?

This is much the same story that we have heard with many murder-suicide and mass murder cases. The warning signs, sometimes not obvious to the casual onlooker, were, nevertheless, there. In February 2012, victim Jackie Wisniewski, who had a long-standing relationship with her killer, went to the West Seneca police voicing her worries about a number of threatening phone calls she had received from her estranged boyfriend, Dr. Timothy V. Jorden Jr. In fact, the threatening phone calls were part of a larger pattern of harassment after Wisniewski, a secretary on the psychiatric ward at Erie County Medical Center, broke up with Dr. Jorden. She couldn't shake him off. Jorden was psychopathically possessive, regarding any woman he came in contact with as his property until he chose to let that property go. That was why, perhaps, at least one element of Jorden's harassment and stalking of Wisniewski involved placing a GPS transmitter on her car. He wanted to know—and let her know that he would know—where she was at all times. If he couldn't have her, nobody would. There would be no escape.

Timothy Jorden's behavior was scary enough. But what was even more frightening about the threats he was making was that he had the capability of carrying them out because he was not just a trauma surgeon. Timothy Jorden had been a member of the United States Army Special Forces, the elite combat unit schooled and trained in the practice of methodical killing. Dr. Jorden was a Green Beret, and that made his mental collapse following Jacqueline Wisniewski's rejection all the more menacing.

Murder victim Wisniewski was certainly not Jorden's only victim in April; the estranged husband of Jorden's personal secretary at Erie

County Medical Center complained to Jorden's employer that Jorden was behaving in an "inappropriate, unethical, and unprofessional" manner towards women who worked with him. Yet despite the complaints lodged with local police, there was no follow up. Jorden, the police said, could have been arrested, charged, and even released with a court order of protection. However, absent any formal charges or a criminal complaint that was actionable, there was nothing between Wisniewski and the person harassing her except time and the seething fury in her killer's mind as he ruminated over what he would do to assuage his anger over being rejected by her.

West Seneca Police Chief Edward F. Gehen told the *Buffalo News* that this was not a case where the victim was at fault. However, many women are reluctant to get the police involved in a relationship dispute. "I'm not blaming the victim; I would never blame the victim," the police chief said. "But we see this way too often with domestic violence victims," Gehen told the local newspaper. Victims just don't want to see an estranged husband or even a boyfriend arrested— or, more often the case, they are rightfully terrified of retaliation once released, as the men often are. According to police records, Wisniewski told them that Dr. Jorden made harassing telephone calls to her, and that he indicated to her that he had knowledge of many of her travels. After that, police discovered a GPS device attached to her car that they believed Jorden had attached so that he could keep track of her whereabouts.

"Our people interviewed her, took a report, found the GPS device on her car, and confiscated the GPS," Gehen said. "Our family offenses detective told her how to apply for an order of protection," the chief explained but added that she never applied for one. Moreover, the police revealed, Wisniewski made only one complaint, but never alleged any violence perpetrated by Jorden against her. Hence, the police, although they were aware of the Wisniewski complaint, had no cause to arrest or to act. Absent a probable cause to open up an investigation, Gehen said that he believed the police handled the complaint properly, although he wished that Wisniewski had filed formal charges so the police could have at least obtained an order of protection for her. When a victim goes to court to seek an order of protection, it requires that the police intervene with an abuser, and a victim's life can be saved, Gehen said. "It should be standard procedure in any harassment situation, especially if the harasser is actually stalking or threatening to stalk the victim. It can save lives because most police don't have the capacity to understand what's in someone's mind or predict what a person will do until that person commits a crime." But, as forensic expert and Bellevue, Washington, Police Chief Donald Van Blaricom (retired) repeatedly stated in these cases, "The victim is often doomed. The police cannot protect her."

Tracy Myles, who alleged publicly that Jorden had affairs with his estranged wife and other female co-workers, said he believes that had more action been taken on a complaint he made to an official of the medical group that employed Jorden, there might have been some intervention on the part of public safety services. Jorden's behavior was unprofessional at best and a red flag at worst and should have indicated that there was potential for trouble.

Myles said he had gone public concerning his contact with the medical group to which Jorden belonged so as to provide notice to the Wisniewski family of his prior warning. In other words, if the medical group at the University of Buffalo or Erie Medical Center had notice of their employee's bad behavior, perhaps the Wisniewski family—and in particular, Jackie's four-year-old son—might have a claim against the Erie Medical Center. Myles said that his email and phone records, "which show Dr. Jorden was in contact with my wife," might provide a basis for their consideration of legal action against Jorden's employer.

As we have learned from scores of mass murder cases and murder-suicides involving workplace and schoolyard locations, if the offender's employer—in this case, Dr. Timothy Jorden—had responded to the complaints about Jorden's womanizing that Myles brought to them in April, things might have turned out differently. Perhaps Wisniewski might have been spared, because Jorden's employer would have intervened and the spotlight would have been placed on him. At least that's the theory. Had Dr. Jorden, because of the focus and the complaints that Myles raised, been placed under scrutiny by authorities, he might have simply fled. However, what we have also found is that murder-suicide offenders—although many try to operate in stealth—also see public identification of their behavior as a precipitating issue that triggers violence. One only has to look at the Jared Loughner case in Tucson to see how identification by authorities can drive an already mentally ill, likely offender further into his madness and derivative criminal behavior.

An exchange of phone conversations and emails between Myles and the University of Buffalo Medical Center, where Dr. Jorden had an affiliation, was also very revealing because it demonstrated that even when a red flag communication was brought to the attention of an employer in authority over the subject employee, sometimes the employer simply doesn't follow through for a number of reasons, including the perceived bias of the individual raising the red flag. In this case, Myles said that in April, he spoke over the phone with Rosemary Boerschig, who was the patient care manager for surgeons at UB/MD. In their call, Myles told the newspapers, Boerschig asked him to send her an email specifically detailing what he told her about Dr. Jorden. She said, according to Myles, that his complaints about Jorden would be sent to the "appropriate people."

On April 23, Myles emailed Boerschig, describing his allegations of an affair between Jorden and his wife, from whom he was estranged and on the path to divorce, and asked the Medical Center to intervene to stop it because his children were involved. The email read: "Dear Ms. Boerschig, I am writing you this letter in regards to the inappropriate, unethical, and unprofessional relationship that has been ongoing between my wife, Colleen Myles, and Tim Jorden, one of your physicians on staff at UB Surgeons. This started two years ago when I noticed a large number of phone calls and after-hours texting between my wife and Tim Jorden."

It was for his children's sake, Myles continued, that he wanted the behavior to stop. "I don't want this to seem as though I am a disgruntled soon-to-be ex-husband. It's for the emotional security of my sons ... If I have to take legal action against Tim Jorden personally, I will. If I have to take legal action against UB Surgeons, I will, along with ECMC. I don't want this matter to further escalate because UB Surgeons and ECMC haven't monitored or care about the quality, character, class, or ethics you have on your medical or office staff."

Responding to the *Buffalo News*, which covered the story of Jorden's murder-suicide and the complaints against him, Rosemary Boerschig was quoted by the News as saying, "I don't want to hear what he has to say. I have no comment."

Colleen Myles said that she told her estranged husband, Tracy Myles, that during the very period when the two were trying to reconcile their marital differences, Jorden had been romancing her and getting in between their relationship. Colleen Myles worked on the third floor of Erie Medical Center's K. Miller Building where, in the basement stairwell, Dr. Jorden shot Wisniewski. For her part, Colleen Myles referred to Tracy Myles as "bitter and disappointed," saying that she felt "the deepest empathy" for both the families of Jackie Wisniewski and Timothy Jorden. She said that she and Jorden had a "personal relationship and worked well together," according to the *Buffalo News*. She did say that she and Dr. Jorden often communicated, primarily because she was his secretary and for that reason he would have had her mobile phone number and would have texted and called her as necessary.

Tracy Myles had an order of protection filed against him by his wife, he said, because he was "inflamed" from time to time at Jorden's intrusion into their marriage. He also said that he was charged with criminal mischief, a case which is pending, because of an argument with relatives after Colleen refused to let him see his sons on Father's Day, even though the visit had already been scheduled. How the claims and counter claims between the Myles's bear on the truth regarding the behavior of Dr. Jorden and the murder of Jackie Wisniewski has yet to be determined, because, in cases of bitter divorces, the truth is often sublimated to the emotional issues of the divorce.

The larger issue, the murder-suicide, raises the all-important question: How could heroic soldier-surgeon Dr. Timothy Jorden become so sick and go berserk? Was it his military experience, or was it a preexisting condition exacerbated by his Special Forces training in the military? Or was it something else; something that clicked in Jorden's mind, telling him his planned escape and disappearance wouldn't work? Did he have to die?

Police speculate that Jorden had not initially planned to commit suicide, although it took him less than an hour to isolate himself and end his life. This might have been why Martin Motley showed up at his house almost immediately after the murder. In the days before the shooting, Jorden pulled $30,000 out of his bank account—presumed to be cash that would support him while he evaded police and tried to start a new life, perhaps with a different identity. He also gave what might be described as parting gifts to his closest friends, and he also seemed to secure an escape vehicle that was not one of his four cars. It was that vehicle, police speculated, that Jorden used to escape the murder scene and perhaps used to drive away while the police put out wants and warrants on one of his registered cars. And perhaps he had relied on Martin Motley, his old high school friend, for help. But that plan changed as Jorden fled from the murder scene and made the decision not to escape, but to commit suicide.

Timothy Jorden's background indicated that he was a planner and could work within the rules of institutions. He joined the National Guard when he was still in high school and entered the Army after graduation, trained for and earning his Green Beret. In Special Forces he was initially a weapons expert, and then his MOS was changed to medic. Jorden completed college and then medical school, earning an officer's commission. Still in the Army, he was sent to Madigan Army Medical Center to complete his training as a surgeon. But shortly after being promoted to captain, he was discharged from the army for either disciplinary or medical reasons that are, at the time of this writing, yet unknown. He was somehow able to complete his surgical training in a civilian training program and became board certified by the American College of Surgeons. He returned to Buffalo to join the staff of Erie Medical. Yet for all his accomplishments, his reported success as a surgeon, and his service to his country in the Special Forces, clearly there was something dreadfully wrong.

Suicide is one of the leading causes of death in the United States and worldwide. Its annual occurrence is approximately twice that of murder. Buffalo's seemingly successful trauma surgeon and highly decorated Special Forces soldier and medic did both. He committed a murder—likely premeditated, since he brought a gun into the hospital—and then found for himself a secluded spot, where he committed suicide. We suggest that trauma was at the root of his mental state of murder-suicide, something we term "mental state of unremitting human destructiveness." For clinicians to try and parse the term "dangerousness to self and others" is to construe a legal construct, oftentimes at odds with the laws of nature. It is a term reserved for both lawyers and doctors acting in a legal capacity on behalf of the court. However, no matter how clinicians or lawyers argue the term "dangerousness to self and others," what psychiatrists know is that there is no one more dangerous than a suicidal person.

A suicidal man has nothing to lose. That was law enforcement's immediate concern when briefing the press on the shooting death of Jackie Wisniewski at Erie County Medical Center. Even Jorden's ex-wife was notified in Tacoma, Washington, just in case he attempted to take her with him in his revenge on those who challenged and then eluded his possessiveness. Authorities were placed on alert due to the ease of his crossing the border into Canada from Buffalo.

When his body was discovered in thick brush on the high bank waterfront of Lake Erie, authorities essentially went mute. At that point, they believed he had only intended to kill one person. But until then, they knew from his military credentials as a Special Forces soldier that he was extremely dangerous, particularly for anyone happening to stand in the way of his secret mission—mad as it was—for escape and revenge. So what drove a man with such publicly recognized strength and fame to the depths of despair? For an answer, we must examine the very personal roots of trauma on human beings who become violent to others and/or commit suicide. When we examine them in Dr. Jorden, we will better understand the epidemic of Post-Traumatic Stress Disorder, and the assaults, homelessness, incarcerations, and suicides in the nearly three million soldiers and veterans returned home from multiple deployments in the war on terror.

We suggest that, to understand what might have driven a highly trained individual such as Timothy Jorden, we have to view "mental states of unremitting human destructiveness," whether to self or to others or both, from the perspective that traumatic events in Jorden's past created a neural response pattern. This pattern was likely exacerbated and made legitimate at the same time by his Special Forces training, and then completely camouflaged by his surgical training. Then it exploded when a woman he considered his personal possession rejected him. It was more than just a blow to his ego. It was a direct threat to his perception of himself that was probably hard-wired—a perception within a damaged psyche in the process of repair to a state of functionality from traumatic damage done to him in childhood. There is both an abnormal psychology and psychobiology to this process of childhood psychological trauma and counter-reparative processes.

In thinking about the possible sources of Dr. Jorden's violence against a loved one, we can look for some clues in the research undertaken by Dr. Felicity Zulueta, who has studied the effects of early childhood trauma on the adult survivor of such trauma. She has been able to penetrate the earliest emotional memories of childhood trauma that occurred, for most part, before her patients had acquired language to tell her what happened. Her test is the Traumatic Attachment Induction Test (TAIT), which can elicit emotional memories that are later translated into language and which tap into traumatic memories of childhood occurring too early for words to convey them. She is able to get her adult patients, many with histories of severe violence and physical harm to themselves, to begin to think about their "representational models of themselves in relation to their caregivers." Dr. Zulueta's research profiles the striking association among childhood abuse, adult violence, and other psychiatric and medical/surgical diseases. In effect, Dr. Zulueta provides a roadmap from adult behavior to childhood abuse or trauma. She also provides case examples of therapeutic use of the TAIT to elicit emotional memories of such abuse to allow patients to reconstruct their internalized representations of both bad parenting they experienced and healthier attachments they did not receive as children. Although we have no direct evidence that Timothy Jorden was abused by his parents, Jorden's psychotic break and his behavior towards colleagues, employees, and patients bespeaks evidence that he was traumatized in childhood, a trauma that may have predisposed him to the effects of adult Post-Traumatic Stress Disorder. Clearly, in retrospect, one can see that he had severe attachment issues.

"The importance of childhood trauma in the genesis of violence and adult ill-health in general can no longer be ignored. The Adverse Childhood Experience (ACE) study carried out in the United States showed that adverse childhood experiences (such as emotional abuse, neglect, and family dysfunction) were much more common than previously acknowledged, and that they have a powerful relationship with ill health 50 years later."[15]

The results of the ACE study are very compelling. Of 17,337 adults responding to a questionnaire-based preliminary study, 11

---

[15] Felitti et al, 1998

percent reported being emotionally abused as a child, 30.1 percent reported physical abuse, and 19.9 percent reported sexual abuse. In addition, 23.5 percent reported being exposed to family alcohol abuse and 18.8 percent to mental illness; 12.5 percent witnessed their mothers being battered, and 4.9 percent reported family drug abuse. The study confirmed earlier research showing a highly significant relationship between adverse childhood experiences and depression, suicide attempts, domestic violence, cigarette smoking, obesity, and sexually transmitted diseases. In addition, the more adverse the childhood experiences, the more likely a person was to develop heart disease, cancer, stroke, diabetes, fractures, and liver disease. Physical symptoms notwithstanding, however, some of the real damage done was social damage, causing an inability to interact with society or authority. According to Teplin et. al. (2002), individuals with childhood histories of trauma make up almost the entire criminal justice population of the United States. This is a staggering statistic almost routinely underappreciated by the public safety and public health communities.

A community-based longitudinal study carried out by Johnson and colleagues (1999) in the United States showed that children who had been abused and neglected were considerably more likely to have personality disorders and elevated symptom levels during early adulthood. All of this points to the truth that residual effects of childhood abuse and trauma can last well into adulthood and be brought to the surface in acts of violence by various forms of incitement or memory stimulation. Or the violence can be triggered by seemingly unrelated events for which everyone, including the perpetrator, could have no awareness. This bears on the Timothy Jorden case, as it relates to what Dr. Zulueta suggests are forms of insecure attachment to the parent or caregiver in childhood.

Dr. Zulueta's research, which stresses that the nature of the childhood's attachment to a caregiver may define the way the adult relates to others, may also seem as though the pop psychology cultures of the 1970s and

'80s have returned, but there is a difference here. This is not about the primal scream, hot tubs at Esalen, or transactional therapy to reach one's inner child. This is about brain function and how, specifically, a childhood trauma might linger like a dormant pathogen within the neurocircuitry of a potential offender, only to be triggered into pathological behavior by an external event for which the offender cannot make any conscious connection. In Jorden's case, the trigger was the emotional devastation of rejection by a woman he believed he possessed. If Charles Swann's visceral memories of childhood, in Proust's Remembrance of Things Past, could be triggered by the taste of a madeleine pastry, imagine Timothy Jorden's visceral memories of loss of attachment—something he could not bear, because it was an existential threat to his core perception of self—being triggered by the rejection of Jackie Wisniewski.

According to Dr. Zulueta, the challenge facing therapists and researchers involves understanding biologically how child abuse can lead to violence and other psychological and physical abnormalities, even if the psychological abnormalities are not apparent, and as with Dr. Jorden, defy the light psychological screening used for checking soldiers' states of mind when returning from war. The root to this understanding lies in qualifying the effects of violence on the brain, particularly the developing brains of vulnerable children in the first two years of life.

Attachment theory and research provide an important psychobiological framework for understanding how environmental experience can trigger both gene expression and developmental outcomes. Human infants are genetically predisposed to want access or proximity to an attachment figure, particularly when they are frightened. We owe this information to Bowlby (1969, 1973, 1980) and his followers, who made the links between human infantile behavior when separated from their caregivers, and the separation studies carried out by ethologists (scientists studying animal behavior) such as Harlow (1974). The latter showed that the longer and the earlier monkeys were separated from their mothers, the more antisocial their behavior in adulthood. Now apply this to children in some single-parent homes, children who spend more time with non-parental caregivers than with their parents, or children placed in an assembly line of foster homes, where any attempts at attachment are tenuous at best, and one can see the problem.

Neuropsychiatric research provides evidence that the psychobiological substrate of attachment behavior in humans involves a great part of the right hemisphere and the supra orbital area of the brain; these very brain regions impaired by childhood trauma are important in the empathic perception of other human beings. As humans are totally dependent on their caregivers in early life, any threat to their sense of security will translate into activation of the attachment system with the characteristic sequence of behaviors: protest, despair, and detachment.[16] Human infants cannot regulate their arousal and emotional reactions, gratify their emotional needs, or maintain psychophysiological homeostasis. As a result, a sensitive caregiver will, in addition to providing protection for the infant, allow for the development of psychobiological attunement between infant and caregiver; a process that provides, from birth onwards, a matching of inner states between mother and infant described by Stern as "affect attunement."[17] The caregiver responds to the infant's signals by holding, caressing, feeding, smiling, and giving meaning to the infant's different experiences. These daily interactions provide the memories that the infant brain synthesizes into "internal working models".[18] These are "internal representations" of how the attachment figure is likely to respond to the child's attachment behavior.

The development of the secure attachment at the same time becomes the representation of the infant's sense of self, which will develop closely intertwined with this "internal representation" of the attachment figure(s). If a satisfactory attunement takes place between

[16] Bowlby, 1970
[17] Stern, 1985
[18] Bowlby, 1988 pp129–33

caregiver and infant, this experience will translate into a sense of security for the child, whose mental representation will evolve into that of a caregiver who is responsive in times of trouble. Such a child will feel confident and capable of empathizing with others, thereby forming good attachments. According to Schore, "this type of attachment becomes a primary defense against trauma-induced psychopathology in later life." We can see manifestations of attachment and non-attachment personalities even in children interacting socially in nursery schools. It is apparent even by age three.

There's another component to this from a biopsychological perspective. Because human beings are one of the few species whose nervous systems develop post-natal, external stimuli (particularly skin contact) arouses the sensors in the infant's skin and transmits those pleasure sensations to the developing brain. Thus, the child experiences basic visceral pleasure and security while it experiences physical boundaries between the self and others. These physical boundaries also enable the child to develop psychological and social boundaries between the self and others—boundaries which, if not developed, can lead the individual to behave antisocially in later childhood. In extreme cases, the individual can develop narcissistic behavior, a dangerous pathology. Extreme narcissistic personality disorders recognize no boundaries between the self and others. They assert ownership or possession of everything in their close interpersonal environs and will destroy the object or person that seeks to defy such sociopathic narcissistic possession. For example, imagine very young children in a nursery school setting. As they interact, even at early ages, you can see which children interact well with others and share, which go off by themselves and have to be encouraged to interact by teachers, and which children are clearly hostile when a school item they believe they possess is encroached upon by another child. This setting is like a laboratory of personality. Now imagine, without changing the personalities of any of these children, you can project them into the future as adults. These are people you recognize; your neighbors, or perhaps your boss.

To put it in more personal terms, imagine a person standing on your toes. You have to tell him to back up because he just doesn't get it that he's hurting you. It's beyond his comprehension that your space or your person that he's violating has any sanctity whatsoever. Yet the individual standing on your toes has the ability to act like a chameleon, turning himself into anything he believes another person would find non-threatening, so as to get something from that person. And this is how the most severe narcissist lives his life. This is the personality type Dr. Robert Hare describes in his psychopathic checklist: the pseudo person who survives by making others feel the way they want to feel. It is the charming doctor who makes you feel so secure and safe that you sign for surgery, even though you don't need it. Does this sound like Timothy Jorden? It does. Had Dr. Jorden been given Dr. Zulueta's utilization of the TAIT, an assessment of him may have gone something like this:

"Dr. X had done some therapeutic work with 'A', a 43-year-old single man who was imprisoned for killing his mate while out stealing in the countryside. On being interviewed by Dr. X, 'A' gave a history of being 'battered' by his mother when a child. He had admitted that he was frightened of her and had begun to make links between his fear and his violent behaviour. The therapist then said, 'Say your mother was sitting over there, what would you say to her?' The patient replies, 'I'd say, "Mother you can't hit me any more. I am an adult."

"The patient slumps in his chair, looks down, and then brings his hand to his face with an accompanying fearful and wary expression—just like the disorganized infants on the return of their caregiver in the Strange Situation Test as described by Solomon and George (1999 p404).

"The therapist continues: 'And you believe that.'

"'Yes, partly,' replies 'A'.

"Dr. X says, 'You partly believe it, and you partly don't?'

"The patient, still looking fearful, says, 'Yes. I don't know whether I could say it to her.'

"'What would stop you?' asks the doctor.

"'Fear,' replies the big man in front of him.

"'Fear of what? What is she going to do?' asks his therapist.

"'Well, she might get up and clout me.'

"The doctor continues questioning: 'Might she?'

"'A', still appearing fearful, replies, 'Well, she might.'

"Even after admitting that his mother is now eighty-five years old and only 5 feet 2 inches tall compared with his 6 feet, 3 inches tall, when the doctor asks him, 'And she is going to do you an injury, is she?' A replies, 'Oh, she is still lively!' He also admits that he can't disagree with her, let alone hit her. This big man is speaking and behaving like a small boy and, although he does seem aware of the fact that his fear of his old mother is irrational, the reality is that at that moment in time, faced with his imaginary mother, the mother in his head, he can only admit to fear, the fear of a child who is terrified of being battered.

"As it turns out, 'A' battered his mate to death when the latter, who had been out stealing with him, insisted that they spend the night in the comfort of his mother's house and 'mouthed' 'A' when he refused."[19]

Although we have no firsthand evidence concerning the childhood history or the military history of Dr. Jorden, based on his behavior during his surgical career—specifically his attachment issues, harassment of those around him, and final murder-suicide—we can make some educated guesses from a clinical perspective. More likely than not—the evidence-based rule of medical, but not legal, certainty—he was forced out of the army as a result of issues at Madigan Army Hospital, where he was completing his surgical residency. The Army was his primary support system and had

---

[19] Johnson, 1999 pp10–4

rewarded his success as a Special Forces weapons and explosives expert. His only means of recovery from such forced separation, and likely perceived abandonment, was an addictive investment in trauma surgery that provided him with the compensatory idealized ego of a savior. Jorden was known to stay in his office overnight, perhaps terrified of the loneliness of his lakeside mansion. Yet, when faced with the challenges of intimacy, he could not rise above what his inner emotional childhood constructs had programmed into the neurocircuitry of the brain regions necessary for empathy and impulse control. He was god-like in the operating room, but more likely than not, he was also a captive of trauma embedded in his brain neurocircuitry, programmed by whatever issues may have afflicted him in childhood.

If severely psychopathological individuals like Timothy Jorden need an external structure to keep their deepest fears in check, institutions and highly regulated professions within those institutions provide that structure because they become like exoskeletons—psychological exoskeletons—holding the person's psyche together in the face of threatening challenges to the psyche. Hence Dr. Jorden's early enlistment in the army and his reliance on the military for college and then medical school training. Even more important, though, is the heavily rule-bound medical profession he chose, one of complete control over himself and a subject: surgery. If one considers that patients in a surgeon's care may feel they are being consulted with, cared for, and healed, then a psychopath under the guise of benevolence can provide exactly what a patient needs with—as Dr. Hare asserts is the psychopath's most dangerous fault—their uncanny ability to make others feel like they want to feel.

Control is complete; even control over his credentialing hospital, where his medical students publicly went on record complaining of Dr. Jorden's performing unnecessary surgeries. His violations of standards of care in routine surgical assessments were probably beyond ethical violations, if the patients' records can be traced. Medical students were quoted in the *Buffalo News* as saying his professional judgment was so impaired that they were turned off surgery as a career choice. In fact, such public complaints were not ethical ones; they spoke of assault and battery committed on the sick and helpless just to get extra fees, teach procedures, or wow onlookers by doing something new surgically. According to comments by one of his students in the *Buffalo News*, not all his medical students were wowed.

So it might have been with Timothy Jorden, whose army experience exacerbated whatever inner conflicts from childhood that he had and then "rejected" him, forcing him to find and build a new external institutional structure in which to function. Failures in intimate relationships with his ex-wife, his romantic liaisons at work, and finally Jackie Wisniewski fractured that structure.

During the Traumatic Attachment Induction Test, the patient experiences imagined separation from the caregiver. This, in an infant or young child, can be traumatic because it generates fear and near panic, coupled with a sense of urging for attachment. The patient relives this. Thus, the TAIT has turned out to be a powerful diagnostic tool in revealing some of the psychopathology underpinning dysfunctional and violent behavior in individuals with a history of childhood abuse. This test points to the importance of traumatization during childhood and its impact on the way human beings both experience and impose violence as adults.

The tragedy of the murder-suicide of Dr. Timothy Jorden and his ex-lover, Jacqueline Wisniewski, is that both the medical communities of the U.S. Army and Buffalo could not—or would not—see that Dr. Jorden's almost messianic healing powers concealed the darkness of a damaged child who had learned the ultimate skills of killing as a decorated Special Forces explosives expert. As with many soldiers returning from Iraq, Africa, and Afghanistan today, Jorden was a coiled snake that, in this case, lurked beneath his surgical garb and behind the wheels of all those fancy cars. And, as his once-manicured lawn turned to weeds and he noticeably declined in physical health, only Officer Motley was there to keep that snake from striking. But what police investigators must determine is whether Officer Motley was more in complicity with the snake than Dr. Jorden's ideal mask of sanity.

Now assume that Dr. Jorden did serve in combat, either as a warrior or medic. More likely than not, his psychological constructs for protecting him from Post-Traumatic Stress Disorder were already askew. Children of abusive families already show abnormalities of brain structure and function before adulthood. So, when they go to war, they are more at risk for developing PTSD.[20]

One clue to the background of Timothy Jorden, the affluent and respected surgeon, was his father's financial situation. Jorden's father lived on the edge of poverty in the very same area where his son grew up. The father was on food stamps, according to the local paper, and did not enjoy the benefits of his son's success. Was this payback? Was Timothy Jorden separating himself from a parent he might have viewed as abusive, and who might have inflicted the kind of traumatic stress on the child that resulted in Jorden's antisocial and ultimately homicidal and suicidal behavior? We don't know. What we do know is that for one reason or another, after becoming the recipient of medical training at the Army's expense at Madigan Army Medical Center in Tacoma, Washington, Dr. Jorden was separated from the military and had to find his own way to obtain his medical license and set up practice in Buffalo. His Special Forces training, far from turning him into a surgeon on a rampage, provided the institutional training that allowed him to subsume whatever traumatic fears he experienced in childhood into a highly rigid hierarchical universe in which he survived until he reached

---

[20] Liebert, Smith and Holiday, "Prevention of Stress Disorders in Police and Military Organizations", Proceedings of the FBI Behavioral Science Unit Conference on Critical Incident Stress Debriefing, Quantico, VA 1989.

an endpoint. He was promoted from lieutenant to captain while in surgical training at Madigan Army Medical Center.

Dr. Timothy Jorden was a self-made, success-oriented individual who was politically adept and knew how to navigate within the taut bureaucratic confines of Army medicine. He had the right stuff for ultimate promotion; even, perhaps, the right stuff for Surgeon General of the Army. But it was not to be. Like the famous soldier-doctor subject of Ted Allan's *The Scalpel, The Sword*; The Story Of Doctor Norman Bethune, immortalized in stone in Bethune Square of Montreal, there was a dark side to this soldier-doctor. Medical students taught by Bethune's colleagues at McGill Faculty of Medicine know of how this greater-than-life narcissist and enigmatic hero's womanizing compromised the faculty's function. And, like the immortalized hero with scalpel and sword, after promotion to the rank of captain, something must have gone terribly wrong at Fort Lewis, Washington, now Joint Base Lewis-McChord, for Timothy Jorden.

Once in private practice, even within an institutional hospital setting, his old fears emerged and manifested as a violent possessiveness. Was there any way to have intervened in Jorden's life as it headed over the cliff? Was there a point at which some outside entity could have flagged this potentially violent at-risk individual and provided him with at least some insight into what was churning inside him? One has to ask where the red flags were, and how many people saw them and did nothing. Tracy Myles pointed to one such flag. Jackie Wisniewski pointed to another. His neatly manicured lawn going to pot, as he himself was physically going to pot, were powerful red flags. If there were red flags that became evident during Captain Jorden's medical training at University of Buffalo, or his surgical training at Madigan, was he simply chaptered out, separated from the Army so the military could wash its hands of someone who was a potential problem?

Only a full post-mortem investigation, including disclosures by Jorden's friend Martin Motley, will provide a fuller portrait of a man, his life, his homicidal act, and his final suicide. Yet Martin

Motley's punishment of getting docked for four days of sick leave after leaving the confinement of his house—for the first time in three years—is likely to be a lone postscript on the strange case of Dr. Timothy Jorden. It is a strange postscript to a lot of lives ruined, and at least one young mother's simply snuffed out. But people from the Pentagon to Tacoma, Washington, and probably all the way to Buffalo, will likely sit on information that could both explain what happened and bring closure. But lest some think that this strange case of Dr. Timothy Jorden was an isolated case, we know that it was not. Unless we understand the brain/mind causality of Post-Traumatic Stress Disorder and other traumatically induced psychological dysfunctions, what might now appear as isolated incidents here and there will become an epidemic of violence. Dr. Zulueta's numbers and thesis, "From Childhood Pain to Adult Violence," both awaken us and make the case.[21]

SOBERING

Once in Vietnam, I saw a boy, sport of our fear, hurled in front of a deuce and a half

When war is over, so is youth and the task of rebuilding for poets and madmen.

But poets commit suicide and madmen go sane, which is, of course, suicide also.

Who notices.

Memorials are a posthumous honor

(Author, anonymous.

Read before Veterans Subcommittee on Oversight by Dr. Liebert on May 2, 1995)

---

[21] (Bethune: The Making of a Hero (1990). The latter, based on a 1952 book *The Scalpel, The Sword; The Story Of Doctor Norman Bethune* by Ted Allan and Sydney Gordon,[28] was a co-production of Telefilm Canada, the Canadian Broadcasting Corporation, FR3 TV France, and China Film Co-production.)

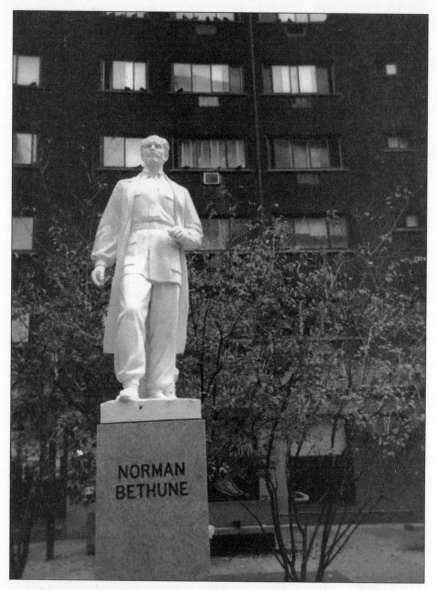

Dr. Norman Bethune's statue in Montreal's Norman Bethune Square.

Chapter 7

Neuropsychiatric Assessment of Psychological Stress and Trauma

The Diagnostic Problems Confronting Military Medicine Today

How do physicians confront the problem of accurately assessing stress and trauma from a psychological perspective? How can physicians make predictions of potential dangerousness and violence? What are the stakes to a physician, to victims, and to the public at large from errors in predicting dangerousness, whether overpredicting or missing dangerousness to self or others? In the face of growing numbers of perpetrators of mass murders and murder-suicides, where does neuropsychiatric assessment of stress and trauma, and the way that stress and trauma combines, form a critical mass of dangerousness that triggers the potential suicidal, homicidal, or murder-suicide patient?

Imagine you are a first-year law student, a 1L, at USC or Stanford. You're taking your torts midterm, and you read the following fact pattern:

Dr. Sy Psychiatrist has been treating Pete Patient, a combat veteran from Afghanistan, in University Hospital's psych ward for eight weeks. Dr. Sy has administered every personality test and psych exam in his repertoire, studied Pete's medical and combat history, and pored over his military and school records. Pete was originally referred to Dr. Sy because he was "acting strangely" and didn't immediately respond rationally to police who'd picked him up for vagrancy months earlier. Pete would soon be automatically released from involuntary confinement at University Hospital if Dr. Sy does not find him dangerous to himself or others.

After six weeks, Dr. Sy believes that Pete does not have a potential for violence. Under the law, he cannot hold him any longer, and he releases Pete into the community.

It takes Pete less than a week to locate his former girlfriend, Gail, and abduct her violently from a bar, drag her into an alley, and stab her multiple times, killing her and then killing himself with the same knife. Police immediately arrive at the scene after neighbors report screams, and they discover the bodies awash in blood. It is a gruesome scene that makes headlines in newspapers the next day: "Combat Vet Released from Psych Ward; Commits Brutal Murder."

Now Gail's parents have filed a suit against Dr. Sy for negligence and malpractice, alleging that Dr. Sy owed a special duty of care to anyone a violent killer like Pete might come into contact with, and that Dr. Sy breached that duty, resulting in Gail's loss of life. They claim that Dr. Sy had "'peculiar ability' in his therapeutic relationship" with Pete that required him to predict Pete's dangerous and homicidal behavior. "Peculiar ability" is the legal term for holding physicians responsible for "knowing" or being in a position where they "should have knowledge" that a child coughing in a certain way has whooping cough, and "controlling" contact of that patient with everyone else by reporting this contagious disease to public health authorities. We call such contagious diseases like whooping cough "reportable."

In three separate answers, write from the perspective of Gail's parents' lawyer, alleging Dr. Sy's liability. Then write from Dr. Sy's lawyer in your client's defense, and finally write your opinion from the perspective of the judge hearing the case as to whether Dr. Sy is liable to Gail's parents for negligence and malpractice.

This is a standard type of essay question that first-year law students might see in a torts exam. But this also goes to the very core of the nature of a psychiatrist's responsibility to predict dangerousness; a key issue when it comes to dealing with combat veterans who might be suffering from Post-Traumatic Stress Disorder.

This is the problem that psychiatrists face (especially psychiatrists working in or for the military) in diagnosing and treating combat veterans, or even serving members of the military for PTSD or any other mental illness that can result in dangerous behavior towards the patient's self or to others. In this chapter, we walk you through that diagnostic process, a best practice for preventing violence by predicting dangerousness.

As difficult and complicated as it is, psychiatrists and clinical psychologists are at the front line of protecting their own patients and the public at large from violence to self and others perpetrated by psychiatric illness. Nowhere is this more pressing an issue than on the clinical staff at military facilities responsible for screening, diagnosing, and treating the usually invisible wounds of war, whether PTSD, post-concussion syndromes of traumatic brain injuries, or impulsive violence or suicidality—all either generated or aggravated by war. What tools do these clinicians have to make predictions of violence to the self, others, or both? In this chapter, we walk through the thicket of psychiatric and clinical psychological screenings and evaluations available to make those decisions, too often with crossed fingers.

Criminologists, psychologist commentators, and many self-proclaimed television pundits who populate the cable news channels have expounded on the nature of homicide, saying that the mass murders perpetrated by Major Hasan, Sergeant Bales, James Holmes, Jared Loughner, and Cho Seung-Hui, or murder-suicides such as the one perpetrated by acclaimed trauma surgeon Dr. Timothy Jorden in Buffalo, are one-off crimes; unpredictable and unpreventable. They are absolutely wrong. Theirs is therapeutic nihilism, because it is clear from all the aforementioned cases that clinicians and responsible authorities, including parents, probably saw red flags loudly flapping in the wind. They just didn't know what to look for, didn't understand the "weird" behaviors they were seeing, or simply chose to ignore them in the hopes that either the behaviors or the people acting weirdly would simply go away. But they don't go away. Instead, they fester, and their mental illnesses begin to metastasize into dangerous and violent ideations.

Statistical rarity of violence of any type in clinical populations does not eliminate clinicians from duty to protect in any one case. Failure to diagnose pulmonary emphysema in a patient with shortness of breath can be malpractice, because doctors know certain patients are at risk for it and can die from it without treatment. Injury from violence to the self is as common as pulmonary emphysema is as a cause of death. Homicide is half the mortality of pulmonary emphysema and suicide. Thus, clinicians cannot be complacent in their decision-making. Yet violent death is different from that of natural disease processes because it leaves in its wake so many loved ones and friends with Post-Traumatic Stress Disorder. Violent death is like dropping a synchronized bomb into the placidity of Walden Pond. The sudden surface waves repeat until eventually diminishing, but they never stop. Similarly with the post-traumatic suffering of loved ones and friends of suicide and homicide victims, the emotional perturbation diminishes, but never goes away.

American law places a burden on clinicians who fail to see potential harm in their patients, particularly when those patients perpetrate violence either under the clinician's care or after having been released from that care under the mistaken belief that the patient is not a danger to the self or others. In what is now controlling law in the state of California, the California Supreme Court reversed a decision absolving University of California clinicians of liability for releasing a patient who presented a danger to his girlfriend, even though these clinicians filed for involuntary commitment of the patient. The Berkeley Police did not think there was probable cause for holding the patient and released him. He hunted his girlfriend, Tatanya Tarasoff, and killed her. The Supreme Court reversed lower court decisions because they deemed that University of California clinicians did not use common sense in both knowing the killer was dangerous and not doing everything possible to protect his girlfriend. They found them negligent in the death of the victim. This is known as the "Tarasoff Decision," which requires clinicians to warn potential victims of potential threats from their patients, just as they would if the patient had a reportable contagious disease. It is the law of the land in California, rightly or wrongly, that clinicians have as much professional responsibility, knowledge, and ability to control many presenting cases of violence to the self and others as they do in diagnosing and controlling patients with contagious diseases.

The chief justice of the California Supreme Court told psychiatrists and psychologists that the Tarasoff Decision was simply a matter of using common sense when having knowledge of patient's dangerousness. It has been proven that 80 percent of completed suicides are by primary care patients who visited their doctors just months before killing themselves and documented a desire to discuss suicidal ideation or urges in that visit. Certainly some of these suicides, therefore, could have been prevented. That is the "common sense" that the Supreme Court of California admonished clinicians to exercise in their practices. A psychiatrist's failure to exercise such common sense in a certain percentage of such cases where the case documentation of a patient is more probably than not predictive of homicide, or constructively by extension, suicide, can therefore be an extreme example of professional malpractice in extremis. The types of evaluations set forth here demonstrate that (without compromising anyone's rights to Fifth Amendment due process or Fourth Amendment protections against search and seizure) medical evaluations can identify, screen, and point to a diagnosis of potential violence, along with suggested triaging procedures and ultimately treatment, in a high percentage of cases. Not in every case, we assert.

Clinicians are not soothsayers by training. But the California State Supreme Court established the bright line: Use common sense, and don't hide behind ethical concerns of patient confidentiality when your patient is clearly going to kill himself or somebody else. A cover with the mesh of privacy rules and regulations justified a sloppy and inadequate psychiatric evaluation of Cho Seung-Hui while he was detained on an emergency seventy-two-hour hold for threats of both suicide and violence, which he ultimately went on to commit. It is this absence of common sense, when knowing a patient is potentially dangerous to the self or others, that Supreme Court Justices were confronting. Not only did Cho's erotomanic target, Emily Hilsher, die, but so did scores of others, along with psychotic Cho himself.

Physicians can, and should, make the necessary assessments. Doing everything by the books and "using common sense" is, according to the California Supreme Court Decision, akin to exercising the "peculiar ability" vested in physicians when examining a child with a whooping-type cough, thus having special knowledge and authority to report the contagious disease to public health authorities. This "peculiar ability" has been transferred over to psychiatrists and psychotherapists, who are expected to know the dangerous outcomes of disease states and prevent them.

Physicians have been classifying the physical and emotional distress of their patients since ancient times. Hippocrates (470-ca.360 BCE), in his discourses on ailments that afflict human beings, classified mental disorders, including paranoia, epilepsy, mania, and melancholia. The historical evolution of this taxonomy—or hierarchical organization of patient "presentations" and "problems"—has resulted in what we call clinical nosology, the formal naming of clinical entities that is the organizational basis of medical diagnostics encoded in the world's diagnostic bible—the International Classification of Diseases, or ICD. This ICD standard statistical manual, recognized among physicians and associated health care clinicians worldwide, classifies clinical entities necessitating encounters with clinicians for diagnosis and treatment. These classifications are based on observable symptoms and signs and are dependent upon either known causation (like tuberculosis), or upon the clarity of diagnostic presentation with reliability and stability of presentation over time (such as coronary artery disease).

Diagnostic "reliability" means that most peer clinicians would agree with the diagnosis, even though all of them could be wrong. "Stability over time" means that competent clinicians are not going to change the diagnosis over and over again. The diagnosis of coronary artery disease informs such costly and potentially dangerous interventions that stability of the diagnosis over time is necessary to avoid unnecessary cardiac surgeries. We now have stent insertions and arterial cameras to view what's going on inside a patient before bypass surgery, so as to avoid opening them up only to discover that he or she is perfectly healthy. Psychiatry is in a state of flux because of recent advances for actually seeing the brain pathology underlying serious mental illness, Post-Traumatic Stress Disorder, suicidality, impending violence, and post-concussion syndrome.

Tuberculosis, heart disease, diabetes, lymphoma, bacterial infections, and varieties of arthritic conditions are all measurable diagnostically because there are physiological manifestations of the pathology that diagnostic testing strongly signals. Because of the controversies over medical effects of stress and trauma evolving from escalating disability claims from both compensable war and civilian traumatic incidents, also known as "critical incidents," it is necessary, therefore, to know how modern clinicians apply diagnostic terms to diseases they diagnose and then code with standard numbers for many purposes. These include insurance billings, medical research, and computerized tracking of a disease course over time on an electronic health record, such as the Armed Forces Health Longitudinal Technology Application (formerly CHCS II, now AHLTA). Longitudinal means that a disease is tracked across its evolution over time, an important component of a permanent health record.

ICD diagnostic terms and their codes change with the times, both through changes in clinical presentations that are little understood (such as chronic fatigue syndrome) or even political in nature (such as Post-Traumatic Stress Injury, considered a replacement for Post-Traumatic Stress Disorder). Policy oftentimes drives reality when disease causation and specific diagnostic testing is either not available or not considered a standard of practice. For example, neuropsychological testing is highly sensitive and reliable in detecting traumatic brain injuries, but it takes a lot of time and resources to do. Had Sergeant Bales received neuropsychological testing, his fitness-for-duty profile would likely have precluded his deployment to Afghanistan, thus preventing the mass murder atrocities. Would that have been worth it? Obviously, and how many more Sergeant Bales fitness-for-duty profiles are dangerously faulty due to a failure to utilize diagnostic testing, like that available for clearing stealth pilots to fly billion-dollar airplanes?

The sophisticated testing performed for selection and maintenance of crew effectiveness on stealth bombers is required for all special ops personnel. The testing to medically clear at-risk Special Forces soldiers sent to remote forward operating bases—like Bales—where they can literally precipitate what might turn into a nuclear crisis, should not be the same as that for pilots, but it must be equivalent, according to the Human Reliability Program (HRP).

The HRP is an enhanced security and safety reliability program designed to ensure that individuals in positions requiring access to certain materials, facilities, and programs meet the highest standards of reliability, as well as physical and mental suitability. Two DOE programs with significant similarities, the Personnel Security Assurance Program (PSAP) and the Personnel Assurance Program (PAP), were consolidated into the HRP by 10 CFR Part 712. The CFR is the Code of Federal Regulations, updates to which are published every day, and which establishes, as a matter of law, how the federal government administers policy. 10 CFR Part 712 establishes a single management structure and a uniform, comprehensive, and concise set of requirements.

Were the regulations as set forth in the HRP consistently applied to combat soldiers deployed to sensitive operations, there would be more scrutiny in assessing the emotional capabilities of those solders and in making predictions of how those soldiers, subject to multiple deployments, would operate under intense pressure. This, of course, applies to Afghanistan and those areas bordering on Pakistan. Pakistan is teetering as our ally and its commitment to secular control of its nuclear weapons. Atrocities like those committed by Bales so close to Pakistan's sensitive strategic border is enough to tip the balance of who is actually in control of this dangerous Central Asian nuclear arsenal.

It is believed that the United States currently has control of the area's nuclear arsenal. But what happens if we are forced out of Afghanistan due to repeated failures in command, a failure in force health protection due to inaccurate fitness-for-duty exams at home bases, and a lack of adequate forward medical support, including psychiatric support in combat theaters and insufficient force protection due to zero-defect security screening of Afghan soldiers. Losing that control could be catastrophic for the entire region, including the United States and her allies. Diagnostics, therefore, are of such critical importance for the human reliability of our armed forces in the nuclear tinderboxes of this world that the military should be required to test its special operations personnel operating with such freedom from command—as was the case with Bales—utilizing thorough testing similar to that used for pilots of billion-dollar bombers. It is the law to remove impaired soldiers. Sergeant Bales would certainly not have met the standards of human reliability under the law and should have been removed long before his last deployment. As set forth in the HRP, there is a formal process to temporarily remove an individual from HRP duties for either a safety- or security-related concern. Temporary removal is not in itself a cause for loss of pay, benefits, or other changes in employment status. The process of removal and appeal is found in the Code of Federal Regulations (10 CFR § 712.19 through § 712.23).

Is such testing too expensive? Too resource-intensive? What kind of war is this; fought on a shoestring budget for clinical resources both at home and in the combat theater? What was the cost benefit of not giving Robert Bales the battery of tests he should have received prior to his fourth deployment—given his known combat-related traumatic head injury, his Post-Traumatic Stress Disorder, and his partial foot amputation—against the payments made to the families of Bales's victims? As high as that total may become, solace payments made to surviving families of Staff Sergeant Bales's atrocities ignore the true cost of the disaster caused by his being deployed with seriously flawed diagnostics that generated his fitness-for-duty profile. He was not fit for duty. And, if his fitness-for-duty profile had been diagnostically accurate, his deployment would have required a waiver from Joint Base Lewis-McChord Base Command. According to his attorney, this was not done at Joint Base Lewis-McChord.

What did the atrocities of this diagnostics failure cost? Certainly it would not be an exaggeration to say it cost innocent civilian lives, the lives of our troops, and a corruption of our policy to prosecute a war in Central Asia. Whether negligent or policy-driven, bureaucratic politics influenced the diagnostic coding for Sergeant Bales, as it does for too many other soldiers and veterans. It puts ticking bombs, individuals who should be sidelined from combat, assigned to administrative or training duties or simply treated and separated from the military, back into the very stressful situations that triggered and then exacerbated their disorders. In so doing, the military undermines its own policies to the detriment of its war effort. The Department of Defense simply ignores the standards of its own Force Health Protection.

Diagnostics for Post-Traumatic Stress Disorder, traumatic brain injury, and psychiatric disability on fitness-for-duty exams can be as operationally valid as the Department of Defense demands that they be. But how can the overlap between symptoms of PTSD and TBI be deciphered when neurologists in the TBI clinic cannot get a psychiatrist to see their patients in consultation because there are not enough of them anymore? The psychiatrists left in U.S. bases are bogged down in twenty-four-hour emergency care, oftentimes without the minimal support of a mental health crisis unit in the emergency room. Too many times, in large hospitals with in-house emergency medicine residents in training, psychiatrists are up all night alone when on night and weekend call. At other times, psychiatrists' work is restricted for alleged budgetary reasons. They are not doing their jobs because the bureaucratic demands of their assignments are impeding their ability to practice medicine, specifically the identification, diagnosis, and treatment of military personnel suffering from PTSD. Even worse, since the demoralizing impact of continuing AHLTA failures and the scandal of the Fort Hood shootings, there are fewer and fewer experienced uniformed psychiatrists to lead. The good and experienced are being replaced, often with non-psychiatrists or psychiatrists who either have not or will likely not be deployed. This is not the way to support the troops that are fighting the war and not the way to handle their legitimate psychiatric problems.

PTSD with potential for dissociative breakdowns is more common than most in the military will admit. As is likely the case with Bales, extreme PTSD, where the patient is suffering from a dissociative breakdown, can be detected with solid clinical interviewing, accurate combat history, and use of selective testing, such as Sleep Lab and the Dissociative Experiences Scale. Additional psychological testing in the hands of skilled clinical psychologists can pick up faking symptoms soldiers use to get out of deployment. All the cases of triple and quadruple deployments, at the very least, should have fitness-for-duty exams on record, complete with psychiatric assessments in resultant fitness-for-duty profiles in the electronic record, AHLTA.

The primary question raised in the cases of Bales, Hasan, and Jorden is the same: How were the diagnoses made? Were they made based on purely combat medicine-driven information, or by administrative and political pressures for a particular outcome, perhaps punitive? For example, does the military send Major Hasan and Sergeant Bales to Afghanistan and simply damn the obvious combat disabilities? Discharge Dr. Timothy Jorden for disciplinary or medical reasons?

As Americans who won the Cold War from what President Reagan described as an "evil empire," we must never forget some of the practices—particularly psychiatric practices within Gulag-like, torture-laden mental institutions—that made the U.S.S.R.

evil. To allegedly evaluate a soldier returning from combat with administrative prejudice about his faking symptoms to bilk the system for long-term disability payments is a rebuke not only to that soldier's service—it is also medical malpractice. Such prejudicial attitudes in evaluating soldiers in distress violate Miller's major rule of bad diagnostics: Find the criteria-based symptoms before judging the patient by diagnosing him.

"This is how prejudicial diagnostics corrupted the Soviet practice of psychiatry, and it threatens to corrupt any health care system rewarded for reducing payments for compensation based on diagnostics. In the case of the Soviet Union, diagnostics were to suppress dissent, justified by the basic tenets of Marxist doctrine. There cannot be mental illness in a perfect society, thus the dissident must be crazy."[22]

Unfortunately, under the bureaucratic or institutional pressure of outcome-predetermined diagnosis, even trained clinicians will too often see what they are told to see, and otherwise scrupulous medical evaluators will be forced to succumb to policy when it comes to processing patient claims for compensation. We don't like it, but it's true. Think of policy-determined medical evaluations as the dark singularity at the center of a galaxy around which truth bends. Policy distorts truth and ultimately creates new reality. Wasn't this the treachery known as Soviet psychiatry, against which the Western medical establishment railed? The politically-based Soviet psychiatry dogma said that all those who were dissidents had to be mentally ill. Therefore, psychiatry had a medical and political focus: to turn dissidents into loyal worker-citizens by curing them of their mental illness. This new type of political patient was termed "Homo Sovieticus" by psychiatrist Walter Reich.

We need to bring the best of diagnostic tools and the best of clinicians to our returning soldiers. To do otherwise is not only

---

[22] Reich, Walter, M.D., "Diagnosing Soviet Dissidents," *Harpers,* August, 1978. ibid.

an insult to our soldiers and an entire profession, but an insult to those sacrificing to defeat our nation's enemies. Our soldiers, like their civilian peers, are not diagnosed in a vacuum interspersed with symptoms they bring to a clinical interview. Bringing research to the clinical office affects diagnostics, too. This is called translational research.

For example, it made less difference in the 1960s whether a disorganized psychotic patient was diagnosed with Schizophrenia or Manic Depression because the treatment was the same, specifically either major tranquilizers, like Thorazine, or electroconvulsive treatment, also known as shock treatment. But then the lithium ion was discovered to quiet mania, and treatment options began to change. When the FDA approved lithium for treatment of mania in 1970, it became critically important to differentiate psychosis caused by Schizophrenia from that of Mania, because the treatments would be different. Thus did politics and social change influence diagnostics.

The same type of social change and social awareness dramatically affected the official medical view of homosexuality with the elimination of homosexuality as a psychiatric disorder. But despite the apparent troubled waters of psychiatry, there is a counterthrust of renewal, potentially transforming this medical specialty into "brain-based psychiatry." Progress in neuroscience influences diagnostics, as can be seen from the burgeoning findings from brain studies of both the seriously impaired psychiatric patient with serious mental illness that is mainly genetically determined, as well as the combat soldier who simply cannot fight another day.

Medicine and the reporting of medical illnesses are highly organized, categorized, and harmonized within the profession, so that doctors in one country can understand and appreciate the research of doctors in other countries. Medicine has become internationalized. Thus, the International Classification of Diseases (ICD) is designed to promote international comparability in the collection, processing, classification, and presentation of mortality statistics. This includes reporting causes of death on the death certificate. The reported conditions are then translated into medical codes through the use of the classification structure and the selection and modification rules contained in the applicable revision of the ICD, published by the World Health Organization. These coding rules improve the usefulness of mortality statistics by giving preference to certain categories, both by consolidating conditions and systematically selecting a single cause of death from a reported sequence of conditions. The single selected cause for tabulation is called the "underlying cause of death," and the other reported causes are the non-underlying causes of death. The combination of underlying and non-underlying causes is the multiple causes of death. In regard to psychiatric diagnostics, the ICD has been revised periodically to incorporate changes across the entire medical/surgical field. To date, there have been ten revisions of the ICD.

For many physiological medical issues, doctors follow specific guidelines established by their respective professional medical communities. For example, a patient walks into a doctor's office complaining of frequent urination, a dry "cottony" mouth, and a thirst that simply will not go away. You take the blood pressure and heart rate, both of which are high. You order a blood test and the results come back with an A1C, an average of the sugar surrounding red blood cells, of a 7.5. Too high. You notice that the bad serum cholesterol is very high. You now have the triple threat for heart disease: diabetes, hypertension, and high cholesterol. You know immediately that your patient should take full dose aspirin—a blood thinner—for at least six months. You will drop it to a lower dose later, but preventing a first heart attack is your major concern. You may prescribe a statin such as Lipitor to reduce cholesterol and perhaps a beta blocker, like Coreg, to help control blood pressure. You put the patient on a low-carb and high veggie diet, tell the patient to add legumes such as unsalted raw peanuts or cashews, drink at least three glasses of water per day, ban all refined sugar, and tell the patient, "This Bud's not for you," thus dramatically curtailing any alcohol intake. And you will probably start the patient on Metformin or Januvia to control blood sugar.

All of the above regimens are standard in the American Heart Association and the American Diabetes Association. You follow them because it's good established medicine that statistics say works. You also follow them because you're careful and know that if you deviate from standard practice and your patient has a fatal (but preventable) heart attack on your watch, you're looking at an expensive medical malpractice suit in which the plaintiff will put an expert witness on the stand who will recite, as if it's gospel, the standard medical practice from which you deviated. So you adhere to standard practice if you want your patient to stay alive, you want to stay out of court, and you don't want your medical malpractice insurance premium to drive you out of the profession.

For overtly visible injuries, we also have basic guidelines. To demonstrate modern taxonomy in medicine, the presenting problem of "burns," our case-in-point example here, serves as a paradigm for more easily comprehending what disease classification is. Disease classification is also known as taxonomy. A presenting problem like "burns" means that this is the problem that the patient presents to a physician—usually to an emergency room physician. The following graphics and charts exemplify the procedure for classifying the type of burn a patient presents and the triaging of that patient in a treatment queue from immediate/urgent life-saving treatment to taking other patients first who present more life-threatening symptoms. We then apply this protocol to psychiatric problems with a specific eye to diagnosing for dangers to the patient's self, to medical staff, and to others.

The cause and appearance of burns are both hard fact. And burns, like coronary artery disease, have a high degree of clarity that informs best practices for clinical management. In other words, we know what causes burns and we know what they look like. Juxtaposing the clinical presentation of a person injured by stress or psychological trauma to the clinical presentation of burns, we are oftentimes struck by the lack of obvious impairment in the former compared to the latter. Clinicians oftentimes refer to such diagnostic dilemmas as "hard" versus "soft" diagnoses, respectively. The lack of clarity becomes evident in international studies. We can make reliable and valid statistical comparisons of burns in Singapore and the United States. But we cannot do the same with psychic injury caused by stress or psychological trauma due to the differences in national and cultural definitions.

Pulmonary tuberculosis, for example, presents itself with typical signs of productive cough that contains the tuberculous bacillus—which, after microscopic examination of the sputum, provides a "hard" diagnosis. Post-Traumatic Stress Disorder and other stress disorders are more arbitrarily defined by specific criteria in the patient's history (such as nightmares of the actual traumatic incident) and are oftentimes called—like fibromyalgia and chronic fatigue syndrome—a "soft diagnosis" by most doctors, including psychiatrists. A soft diagnosis is subject to both excessive sensitivity to interpreting patient's history, and of most importance, judging the severity of psychological trauma, as is necessary in evaluating patients after an auto accident or rape. Conversely, the diagnosis of PTSD is subject to excessive rigidity in eliciting and documenting necessary symptomatic criteria to meet the diagnosis. In the former case, there is a risk that stress and Post-Traumatic Stress Disorder will be overdiagnosed, while in the latter, there is a risk of it being underdiagnosed. Many Holocaust survivors, for example, are so emotionally shut down—or numbed, as a means of surviving death camps—that they will deny nightmares. In fact, often they either do not dream at all or do not recall their dreams. It is a defense mechanism; a protection of the self from the unspeakable horror—a horror beyond any imagination—that they suffered. A survivor's failing to recall dreams promotes his or her functioning during the day, instead of setting off a chain reaction of the debilitating reliving of camp memories and the sadness—the deep, penetrating sadness that would never abate.

Lacking standardized and validated objective testing for the pathological impact of stress and psychological trauma, controversy over diagnosis emerges when monetary considerations come into play as result of damages from war or second party or defendant liability, as in an auto accident. Accordingly, it is important for us to ascertain how such traditional clinical perception of "softness" in diagnosis plays out in escalating controversy over compensable wounds of war. Compensable wounds are wounds doctors can see, like bullet wounds and burns. For example, Post-Traumatic Stress Disorder alone does not qualify a soldier for a Purple Heart, whereas a shrapnel wound received in combat does. A Purple Heart is awarded only in the case of visible physical wounds of war; the argument against the award for Post-Traumatic Stress Disorder is its apparent invisibility. A more sinister explanation, perhaps, is the soldier's own weakness or failures in the combat situation.

The dichotomy between visible and invisible wounds comes right out of the scene from the film "Patton," where the general did not consider combat stress be a true combat wound. This dichotomy, however, is now disappearing because of the emergence of new technologies to make the formerly invisible now visible. Post-Traumatic Stress Disorder (like chronic fatigue syndrome), traditionally known as a soft diagnosis subject to different interpretations from different clinicians, is not soft anymore because of established, thorough, criteria-driven diagnostic interview and collateral testing.

We can provide clear and convincing evidence beyond the usual standard of medical evidence that Post-Traumatic Stress Disorder is a now hard diagnosis, visible with new sleep and imaging studies in support of thorough skilled interviewing and psychological testing.

This means the standard called diagnostic specificity, separating the symptoms of PTSD from all other psychiatric disorders presenting with similar symptoms, like social isolation and avoidance, panic attacks, and insomnia. Diagnostic specificity that separates those with partial syndromes from malingerers faking symptoms for compensation is therefore improving, but the testing is complicated and expensive, thus limiting its translation from research to Army and VA clinics. Such application of research and development from lab to practice is called translational research, which, we believe, is the core of a new medical frontier when it comes to traditionally soft diagnoses that, like combat-induced PTSD and TBIs, can be so disabling and potentially lethal to the patient or those he comes in contact with.

The multiaxial diagnostic template known as DSM IV refines the taxonomy of ICD through a comprehensive nosology, or naming of presenting clusters of symptoms, designed to capture all clinical encounters with mental disorganization and emotional distress. It therefore captures most of the robustly symptomatic cases of Post-Traumatic Stress Disorder. The criteria required for a clinician to make the diagnosis of PTSD are as follows:

A. The person has been exposed to a traumatic event in which both of the following have been present:
    1. The person experienced, witnessed, or was confronted with an event or events that involved actual or threatened death or serious injury, or a threat to the physical integrity of self or others.
    2. The person's response involved intense fear, helplessness, or horror. (Note: In children, this may be expressed instead by disorganized or agitated behavior.)

B. The traumatic event is persistently reexperienced in one (or more) of the following ways:

1. Recurrent and intrusive distressing recollections of the event, including images, thoughts, or perceptions. (Note: In young children, repetitive play may occur in which themes or aspects of the trauma are expressed.)

2. Recurrent distressing dreams of the event. (Note: In children, there may be frightening dreams without recgnizable content.)

3. Acting or feeling as if the traumatic event were recurring; includes a sense of reliving the experience, illusions, hallucinations, and dissociative flashback episodes, including those that occur upon awakening or when intoxicated. (Note: In young children, trauma-specific reenactment may occur.)

4. Intense psychological distress at exposure to internal or external cues that symbolize or resemble an aspect of the traumatic event.

5. Physiological reactivity on exposure to internal or external cues that symbolize or resemble an aspect of the traumatic event.

C. Persistent avoidance of stimuli associated with the trauma and numbing of general responsiveness (not present before the trauma), as indicated by three (or more) of the following:

1. Efforts to avoid thoughts, feelings, or conversations associated with the trauma.

2. Efforts to avoid activities, places, or people that arouse recollections of the trauma.

3. Inability to recall an important aspect of the trauma.

4. Markedly diminished interest or participation in significant activities.

5. Feeling of detachment or estrangement from others.
6. Restricted range of affect (i.e., unable to have loving feelings).
7. Sense of a foreshortened future (i.e., does not expect to have a career, marriage, children, or a normal life span).

D. Persistent symptoms of increased arousal (not present before the trauma), as indicated by two (or more) of the following:
1. Difficulty falling or staying asleep,
2. Irritability or outbursts of anger,
3. Difficulty concentrating,
4. Hypervigilance,
5. Exaggerated startle response.

E. Duration of the disturbance (symptoms in Criteria B, C, and D) is more than one month.

F. The disturbance causes clinically significant distress or impairment in social, occupational, or other important areas of functioning.

Eliciting these criteria in a well-structured clinical interview should yield few false positive fakes and few false negative misses, particularly if backed up by an intelligent selection of psychological testing. One must always remember the clinical judgment and experience-based expertise required to elicit and observe these criteria in a patient. One must also know that a complex and tight construct for an abnormal clinical state is necessary for research, but it does not necessarily support effective diagnostics informing best clinical interventions. As Dr. Donald Klein states, "For what purpose is differential diagnosis, if not at least partly, to predict clinical course and treatment response?" He further emphasizes the importance of validity in diagnosis along neuropsychiatric clinical pathways.

"The advent of psychotropic drugs has enormously improved psychiatric care ... It has been repeatedly shown that the majority of patients with psychiatric illness go undiagnosed, and even if diagnosed, they are inappropriately or ineffectively treated, both by psychiatrists and primary care practitioners ... The DSM process improved clinicians' ability to communicate with each other by explicit inclusion and exclusion criteria. Nonetheless, our eventual goal is diagnostic validity, which means that diagnoses have practical value. In this context, the use of one diagnostic criteria set rather than another should lead to a superior ability to prescribe, treat, and render a secure prognosis. Here there has been only moderate progress. A clinician's problem is deciding what treatments to select for a particular patient and how to do it. Diagnosis alone is not sufficient, although usually necessary."[23]

The current controversies in formulating diagnostic criteria for DSM V demonstrate the need in psychiatry and clinical psychology for more specific criteria in selecting the right treatment. Nowhere is this controversy more evident than in the diagnosis of PTSD. So, for the busy and experienced clinician, using a checklist on every returning soldier presenting in a military or VA clinic is, as Klein states, not the sole solution, although it's a well-intentioned beginning. We believe that there are partial syndromes that require treatment, and to withhold treatment from a soldier not meeting rigid criteria portends many problems down the road when a full syndrome is likely to emerge, especially if what emerges is a syndrome that manifests a threat to the sufferer's self and others. Thus, better to treat early, rather than wait for the soldier or vet to meet the full criteria, particularly knowing that most of the highly publicized suicides occurring in returning soldiers and vets have not been seen by a military or VA clinician.

---

[23] Klein, D., et. al., Clinical Psychopharmacological Practice, The Need of Developing a Research Base, *Arch. Gen., Psychiatry* 50, 1993

In contradistinction to this clinical course of a disease, most completed suicides are preceded by a visit to the victim's primary care provider within months of death and with documented desire to talk about intense suicidal urges. The question is, why the difference between soldiers and veterans completing suicides and their civilian peers?

Paul Miller wrote that paying attention to diagnostic criteria may not, as Klein states, help in selecting specific treatment, but it does lead to what is known as diagnostic reliability. Diagnostic reliability means that most clinicians evaluating the same patient for the same presenting complaints are consistent with addressing the DSM criteria. Paul Miller's research at UCLA teaching hospitals shows a consistent mismatch among different clinicians evaluating and treating the same patient for the same symptoms within a short duration of time. This is also common in the military, as demonstrated on the electronic health record known as Armed Forces Health Longitudinal Technology Application, or AHLTA. The soldier's treatment is both delayed and misguided by numerous clinicians calling "the problem" something different. For example, the medic might call it an "occupational problem with insomnia" during a combat mission, while another clinician might call the same symptoms depression.

With such a panoply of different causes parsed into it for the same problem in the same patient by different clinicians over time, "longitudinal" becomes self-defeating because the complexity makes it meaningless. When it comes to validity and specificity of diagnosis, one can often object anecdotally to what AHLTA's problem list shows. Going only by that problem list, any clinician might simply say, "If it looks like a duck, talks like a duck and walks like a duck, it is a duck." The problem is that's not always the case. Therefore, even though there may be different diagnoses, balance is needed between Klein's emphasis on treating the patient, rather than the cold DSM criteria, while Miller brings attention to a wide scattering of diagnoses in the same soldier for the same presenting problem by different clinicians over time. This problem can be solved now by fixing the military electronic health record that drives so many clinicians out of the Army and drives others still in a bit crazy.

It is important to understand that the diagnostics in PTSD (as in TBI and all other ICD clinical entities) change with both the accelerating growth of clinical literature, as well as hard laboratory evidence in both our civilian population and our nearly 3 million men and women who have been deployed in combat since 9/11. The Army Surgeon General communicated via email to all its doctors that the Armed Forces Health Longitudinal Technology Application was the main reason for clinicians leaving the Army. Rather than complain about the application, the answer is to fix AHLTA. The application can narrow clinician discretion in simply entering problems on a soldier's health record without conforming to diagnostic criteria cited in Paul Miller's studies and diagnostic validity that predicts outcomes with and without certain clinical interventions, as cited in Donald Klein's studies. The mystery remains: why spend billions to modernize AHLTA, without improving its computerized clinical decision support analytic functions? It is a Technological Application. However, few clinicians who have to practice off it in the Army would say it is a very good one. It's a clunker, and everybody knows it's a clunker.

The problem with all diagnostic templates and clinical nosologies for the disease states driving them is that they can dominate both clinical practice and behavioral science investigation. With the advent of promised deliverance from all the woes of current health care through clinical computing, the demands for consistency and simplicity in diagnostic language—or lexicology—now becomes even more important. It is amazing to work within large institutions, and over and over again, see patients carrying multiple diagnoses for the same presenting problems. We work towards inter-rater reliability to harmonize the assessments of symptoms and presentations with diagnoses, but that does not always solve the problem. In fact, it sometimes makes the problem more intractable, because when another medical evaluator comes along, that person must spend time trying to figure out not only the problem the patient may have, but also why the previous medical evaluators couldn't figure it out and came up with different diagnoses.

Recent military medical standards, for example, demanded solid proof of extreme trauma in order to diagnose PTSD. It was the presumed disabled soldier's responsibility to prove extreme trauma on Axis IV. More often than not, it is difficult to get this hard proof, because in the heat of combat, medics are not thinking about how documentation of Axis IV factors is going to affect whether a soldier gets a pension or not when he is out of the Army. He's thinking about getting his patient and himself home alive and in one piece. So this returning combatant will frequently have a string of diagnoses on his electronic health record. They will usually span everything from Occupational Problem, which is essentially interpreted as having trouble fighting; Depression NOS, even though his best friends were just killed; Adjustment Disorder, because he can't sleep before the tenth straight combat mission that month; or Acute Stress Reaction, which is really a factor for Axis IV.

Here is the actual fitness-for-duty profile maintained on all active duty soldiers. Its importance in being maintained is a major subject of what we are addressing. Major Hasan and Staff Sergeant Bales were not fit for duty. How were they profiled as being fit? Both were deployed against their strong personal objections to going into the Afghanistan combat theater.

(Fitness-for-duty profile from Army AHLTA electronic health record. The final letter in the profile, "S," is the military equivalent of the DSM GAF rating on Axis V—thus the numerical rating of either normality of psychological function or impairment.)

The letters "PULHES" refer to the following body parts or organ systems:

"P" – General physical condition, stamina, or any problem not addressed below.

"U" – Upper extremities and upper (cervical and thoracic) spine.

"L" – Lower extremities and lower (lumbosacral) spine.

"H" – Hearing and ear conditions.

"E" – Eyesight and eye conditions.

"S" – Psychiatric conditions.

The electronic health record has significant potential to identify and track epidemiological factors known to either cause or increase the risk of acquiring health problems. Presumably that is why it is called the "Armed Forces Health Longitudinal Tracking Application." These could include monitoring exercise and blood pressure or even life change units that inform patient and doctor to "slow down." Early identification of emotional and physiological breakdown could also help patient and doctor get control of the patient before his psychological train goes off the rails. We need to pick up the suicidal soldiers and veterans who are not currently coming into military and VA clinics for help.

Rare as suicides, homicides, and mass murders on the scale of Hasan and Bales are, their consequences are of such massive scale that preventive measures are necessary. Like episodic killers, suicidal mass killers create a large number of victims relative to their own numbers and singular actions in pulling the triggers. Therefore, we need preventive intervention early. We need to find out what went wrong in the fitness-for-duty examination and clinical monitoring of Major Hasan, Staff Sergeant Bales, violent offenders within the military and VA population, and combat vets at risk for suicide. Unless we know what went wrong, we cannot either prevent disasters like the atrocities of Bales and the Fort Hood shootings of Major Hasan, or maintain force health protection. Without force health protection, we cannot have force protection. That is clearly the lesson of both Bales's and Hasan's cases. And without force protection, we can neither defend this nation in foreign wars nor defend its private citizens inside our own borders.

To complicate matters of military medicine's search for clinical IT solutions, the Diagnostic Statistical Manual is being revised. Will there be pressure to change the nosology—or naming—of PTSD to PTSI to project its essence as an injury rather than a disorder? This could be important from a compensability perspective, because injuries are tangible and visible as opposed to disorders, which the military has heretofore said are not. Regardless of the debate over wording, the inclusion or exclusion of criteria, and the categorizing of its taxonomy as either Post-Traumatic Stress Disorder or Post-Traumatic Stress Injury, DSM needs to meet the demands of diagnostic sensitivity so as not to miss symptoms signaling significant psychiatric illness and abnormal psychology.

For the diagnosis of depression, therefore, DSM must catch all the nuances of "insomnia" so as not to miss one of the critical criteria to make that diagnosis. Absent a diagnosis of clinical depression, antidepressant medication is not indicated. In the cases of both Post-Traumatic Stress Disorder and traumatic brain injury, boundaries for including or excluding a soldier within one or both diagnostic groups can be costly if a soldier is malingering and awarded millions of dollars in long-term disability compensation. Such manipulation of the federal disability compensation system not only wastes taxpayers' money, but it also hardens clinicians into believing they have been conned into destructive diagnostic cynicism. Such cynicism, or diagnostic incompetence, can be deadly if symptoms are missed.

There is no silver bullet test for PTSD or TBI, such as the red blood cell count for anemia. Therefore, there is no substitute for carefully listening to the soldier or significant other's complaints about emotional distress and aberrant behavior with well-timed, empathic questions. A cold, structured interview that inquires about symptoms and signs meeting the criteria for treatable and compensable PTSD or TBI in a traumatized soldier can send him or her running, never to return to any government clinic again. These are patients in a delicate balance. To confront them like a cross-examining attorney trying to prematurely get at their desire to be compensated monetarily, or to seem disinterested in their combat history may smoke out a few malingerers. But the risk of scaring away veterans who are in need of help is too high. Thousands have run from such encounters at the VA, never to return again. Tragically, as resources at the VA are overwhelmed, more are running now and will run in the future. If a soldier is trying to take advantage of the system, this fact will emerge over the course of a proper evaluation that involves regular follow-up appointments and the utilization of supportive psychological, imaging, and laboratory testing.

Disregarding what is known as the therapeutic alliance in favor of a rejection or prosecutorial confrontation promises a low yield for false claims for disability compensation and an extremely high yield of second injuries to wounded minds. Such was a problem in examining survivors of the Holocaust and the concentration on childhood psych problems preceding arrest, incarceration, and torture in Nazi concentration camps. Such focus on problems before incarceration, rather than what happened inside the camps, caused "second injury" by the examining West German psychiatrists entrusted with determining monetary compensation for psychological trauma. Such behavior by German psychiatrists after World War II was reprehensible. Such behavior by military and VA clinicians is equally reprehensible.

The behavior by psychiatric clinical examiners we described above, thankfully, is neither widespread nor tolerated as a standard—but, sadly, it does occur. If the returning soldier or veteran gaining initial access to a military or VA clinic for a psych evaluation is met with apparent disinterest, or worse yet, contempt for presenting a complaint, experiences damaging invalidation that is not dissimilar to that of the incest victim recurrently abused over years without her mother's awareness and acknowledgment. The victim is left to wonder for a lifetime, "Did my mother really not notice my stepdad coming into my room every night, or was she complicit in her denial of my being violated?" Like the Holocaust survivors who were questioned at length about their pre-arrest psychiatric histories to the exclusion of their post-arrest horrors of Concentration Camp Syndrome, both the combat veteran and incest victim are similarly at risk for second injury from clinicians within the uniquely combined disability assessment compensation and treatment environments of military and VA health care.

The nearly three million combat veterans returning or returned from the War on Terror deserve, if nothing else, accurate and valid diagnostics to inform effective clinical interventions. There is no medical reason for not doing this. DSM is not at fault, whether in its current form or a revised form. Within the abnormal human psychological states, known as psychopathology, specific discriminators must serve as tags for meaningful mapping of clinical presentations. The taxonomy of DSM, therefore, must generate a clinical nosology, or naming of conditions, that creates meaningful borders between the normal and abnormal. Presentations signaling either prototypical "mental disorganization" from flashbacks or the classical triage prototype, "strange behavior" from emotional numbing, need to be separated from the dysphoria, or emotional pain, of other conditions with "emotional distress." DSM nosology, therefore, provides clinicians with prototypes subject to more detailed refinement before qualifying to either inform evidence-based treatment of PTSD or qualify a patient for financial reimbursement in long-term disability payments.

Mentally disorganized and strangely behaving patients may neither solicit clinical help nor even have a chief complaint. In fact, statistics on completed suicides among combat veterans returning home demonstrate that the most lethal cases do not get clinical attention. And psychiatrists have seen soldiers with Post-Traumatic Stress Disorder who are, frankly, as delusional as Schizophrenic patients. They will not voluntarily come to a military clinic for assessment because of their delusions. They may live in isolation and merely be seen behaving strangely by others. The emotionally distressed patient seeking relief from mental anguish, however, will feel pain and seek help.

In the following triaging protocol for delineating taxons that are discriminators of "presentations" or "syndromes," the clinician is informed to use caution in an encounter with the person behaving strangely or mentally disorganized without insight into his abnormality. As an example, Dr. Mathew Friedman, director of the National Center for Post-Traumatic Stress Disorders Studies, recently presented a case for the Harvard Psychiatric Academy of a returning female soldier who shocked her neighbors and husband when she showed no emotional response to her young son's near-death experience in an auto-bicycle accident. Patient Sue, when describing this incident, stated that she simply is not herself since returning from combat duty in Afghanistan, because she cannot experience any feelings. She's numb.

"It's not me," she stated. "I wasn't like this before deployment in combat."

In such cases, the emotional numbing is a psychological defense necessary for surviving combat environments without blowing up, but it is abnormal for mothering back home. Carrying that defensive mechanism home after combat to the point where it deadened what should have been a natural parental response indicates that Sue was still reliving the traumatic stress of combat. What once might have been protection was now a severe dysfunction in the world outside of combat. The classification of her presentation should be a red flag to any clinician and needs a disciplined and detailed investigation to diagnose or rule out PTSD.

A patient's emotional distress signals his or her insight into an abnormal state of mind with his or her capacity to communicate for purposes of establishing a safe therapeutic alliance. In other words, emotional distress displayed in an intake or therapy session demonstrates the patient's willingness to discuss what the problem is. This is unlike the former two prototypes cited above that clinically present without obvious distress or insight into abnormal states of mind, specifically the psychotic or primarily numbed patient. Therefore, the clinician has to find other ways to get the patient to relate the nature of the problem. Still, unless the diagnosis informs the clinician of what to do, it is of little pragmatic value in practice. Mood charts show a patient who cannot feel and is therefore tagged alexithymic in mood, which means incapable of feeling emotion. In this case, it is a chronic asthmatic patient who unconsciously and automatically learns not to experience emotion, because laughing or crying bring on asthmatic attacks that prevent her from breathing. Similarly, emotional numbing, as we will later explore in detail, is a protective emotional shield to ward off the overwhelming horrors of combat, but it is devastating to a soldier like Sue who is trying to resume her role as a mother and a wife within normal peacetime circumstances.

STRANGE BEHAVIOR NONVERBAL

1. "May I talk with you?"

   If a patient says "NO" leave area immediately and notify security.

2. Patient considered likely to assault staff. <u>High Risk!</u>

3. If considered that patient is non-combative, notify security, have 4 staff members present and approach patient with caution.

   - Safe eye contact
   - Safe interpersonal space
   - Safe clinician posture
   - DO NOT touch patient
   - Prepare patient for any physical exam
   - Express sympathy
   - Be polite

4. Maintain Airway
5. Maintain adequate breathing
6. Maintain Circulation / Rule out Shock
7. Throw out the <u>W W H H H I M P E S</u>

The current upgrading to DSM V, like the first DSM I of the '60s, is a work in progress. There are many changes being discussed for diagnostic criteria of Post-Traumatic Stress Disorder and Traumatic Brain Injury. Because we rarely know the causation of people presenting clinically with emotional distress, strange behavior, or mental disorganization, it is necessary to categorize presentations into constructs that, first of all, have inter-rater reliability. Inter-rater reliability means that if a patient has multiple medical evaluations by different examining physicians in an emergency room setting, and all the medical evaluations agree on what the problem is, then the presentation of the patient, and the likely diagnosis, has high reliability.

Carrying the concept of inter-rater reliability forward for our purposes in this discussion, therefore, most experienced clinicians agree with the criteria for the psychiatric condition known as Major Depression. Such inter-rater reliability is necessary for researchers and insurance adjusters who have to translate a diagnostic code into monetary value to pay medical or long-term disability claims that oftentimes reach millions of dollars in lifetime benefits.

Reliability, however, does not ensure diagnostic validity. This latter requirement for a meaningful and functional diagnostic system demands that the "entity," or ICD code, informs clinical decision-making from a standard menu, predicting the effectiveness of outcomes and ensuring the stability of that diagnostic name for a condition over time or longitudinally. Simply put, a diagnosis with a five-digit code is of no value if it informs the clinician to order the wrong tests or treatments. And if clinicians have to change the diagnostic label over time as the underlying disease entity evolves, it fails to meet the necessary criteria for diagnostic validity— namely, stability over time. For example, diagnosing a spot on the lung as pneumonia, and then changing the diagnosis to malignant carcinoma of the lung when it spreads to the brain is an example of the treachery inherent in diagnostic invalidity that fails the test of stability over time.

For our specific purposes, it is known that early intervention in the treatment of Post-Traumatic Stress Disorder and Traumatic Brain Injuries reduces the risk of progressive deterioration of the patient, but if that diagnosis is not revisited as the mental illness evolves, it may likely increase the risk of premature death, whether from self-medication via substance abuse, suicide, or psychosomatic complications, such as heart attacks. Therefore, how do diagnostic validity and reliability apply to the equivalent DSM, the operational prototype for directing clinical interventions to reduce the suffering of soldiers and their families following deployment or discharge from the military?

In the case of a DSM prototype with relatively strong evidence-based criteria, we can take the example of an adult patient seeking help for a depressed mood. She meets all the criteria for major depression with insomnia, loss of appetite, lack of interest, and thoughts of suicide. This is the third time such depression has occurred in her life, and there are no other diseases, such as depressed thyroid function, to cause these symptoms. Additionally, there are no other psychiatric disorders, such as alcoholism or other forms of substance abuse, to either cause or correlate with her clinical presentation. Furthermore, she is well-organized mentally, without disordered thinking and abnormal perceptions such as delusions or hallucinations, respectively. Most clinicians will agree that this patient fits the criteria for "Major Depression, Recurrent and Severe, without Psychosis, ICD 9 #296.33." So now most researchers can begin to screen this patient for inclusion in studies of mood disorders, because they all know they are studying the same prototype. But here's the sticky point as it applies to Post-Traumatic Stress Disorder, especially in veterans—how does this inform best practices for treatment?

If suicidal ideation affects proper assessment and safety plan, while the insomnia associated with lack of interest leads to prescription of the antidepressant, Paroxetine, then the diagnosis most likely has high validity, too. Paroxetine will likely be an effective first choice medication for both antidepressant action and nighttime sedation. Its slight adrenergic action could also help improve interest, believed to be dependent on adequate brain adrenalin. If, however, the patient develops panic attacks and total wakefulness over time, the validity of the selection of her original diagnosis as "Major Depression" was poor, because it is not stable over time. The patient has likely become manic, and thus was more likely experiencing Bipolar Affective Disorder, ICD #296.5. With this diagnosis, we could anticipate this patient losing insight during mood cycles and possibly harming or even killing herself. In this case, the diagnosis was sensitive enough to pick up a lethal psychiatric disorder, and it was reliable enough for a multicenter research study.

Everyone involved in a multicenter research project has to agree on what is wrong with all subjects. The diagnosis wasn't valid, however, because it did not predict treatment for effective outcome. Nor was it stable over time. The name of the underlying disordered process had to be changed, totally altering operational demands of clinical management. In fact, it was so unstable over time that the patient might lose insight in a manic state, cycle, and kill herself. The diagnosis of Bipolar Affective Disorder, ICD #296.5, would have been a more valid diagnosis from the beginning, because it would more likely have remained stable over time and even prevented her death. For accuracy from the beginning to have been accomplished, frequently missed states of excitation must be solicited and identified throughout the patient's life. This is hard to do, because the patient may only remember the down times, while forgetting the more energized times, which are oftentimes enshrouded with intoxication or whirlwind activity.

Similarly, we can make the same mistakes in diagnosing Post-Traumatic Stress Disorder, especially if the initial presentation so persuades a clinician that he or she overlooks the possibility that the disease will evolve or change over time. Characteristically, the psychological test profiles of post-traumatic patients show high spikes in psychoticism. Of course, some severe cases of PTSD can in fact be psychotic, as previously cited, with delusions and inability to distinguish external reality from memories of combat both years and thousands of miles away. A returning soldier has often experienced horrors which he or she is afraid to relate to intimates back home for fear of either hurting them or being considered crazy. They feel crazy and show it in answering the questions on commonly used psychological testing with MMPIs. Accordingly, during the immediate post-Vietnam era, VA policy was to dismiss PTSD as a diagnosis because most clinical evaluators saw it as a manifestation of a preexisting psychological condition, and hence, not compensable. This attitude has changed and will continue to change dramatically because of the huge swell of returning veterans, and the realization that the military cannot simply dump sick veterans into the public health and safety systems.

All clinical disciplines seek diagnostic specificity, and the science of modern genetic testing and imaging promise improvements in this requirement for a meaningful and effective nosology. For example, we know that Post-Traumatic Stress Disorder is usually associated with severe nightmares and sleep disorders detectable in sleep lab studies. There is also considerable evidence supporting the theory that PTSD manifests as the phenotype of an abnormal neuropsychiatric genotype timed for vulnerability to trauma at a certain age, as in the young adult soldier. Or the genotype makes a person less resilient to trauma of combat. Accordingly, it would not make sense, for example, to select Special Forces troops from the youth symphony orchestra. It would make more sense to recruit from YMCA boxing rings. If and when we consistently identify the DNA marker for resilience to stress and trauma, something perhaps in an abnormal enzyme assay of serum, and it is consistently correlated with patterns of abnormal regional metabolism on functional MRIs under conditions of stress, we can segregate a large cohort of young adults whose resilience makes them likely candidates for PTSD in combat. Such young adults, paradoxically, may have behavioral problems that are more biologically driven during schooling, but find both the structure and legitimate fighting of military service and combat, respectively, an easier adaptation in life than nursing or engineering careers. Thus, a biological evaluation, should such an evaluation methodology eventually be developed, would be far more valuable for pre-MOS assignment than a simple aptitude test and follow-up interviews. Was this the case of Dr. Timothy Jorden's disastrous transfer from soldier with sword to doctor with scalpel?

Chapter 8

The Madigan Scandal at Joint Base Lewis-McChord

To describe the scandal at Madigan Army Hospital in Tacoma, part of Joint Base Lewis-McChord, is as simple as describing what happens when you file an insurance claim. You go to a doctor with a medical complaint. The doctor makes a diagnosis and describes a treatment plan. Then you file a claim under your medical insurance plan. Once that claim reaches the insurance company, it's reviewed, usually by a doctor in the claims department. That doctor may determine that your claim is valid, and the insurance company should pay. The doctor may—especially if he or she is under the specific instruction to find a way to deny claims whenever possible, because the insurance company wants to find a way out from under the financial burden—deny your claim outright by saying that you are either faking the condition or that the condition is not covered under your policy. If your claim is denied, you can either pay for the treatment yourself or simply not get the treatment, which means the condition may get worse. This, in essence, is what happened at Madigan Army Hospital, where a bureaucracy was set up to deny medical disability claims from soldiers diagnosed with Post-Traumatic Stress Disorder.

Bureaucratic actions, especially in the military and performed for expediency or under pressure, can result in far-reaching and sometimes devastating results. At Madigan Army Hospital, many medical diagnoses were reversed so as to deny soldiers' disability claims. These claims were for mental illness, specifically PTSD claims. In reversing legitimate psychiatric diagnoses for the purpose of denying claims, the special forensic psychiatric unit that was responsible might well have put soldiers back into combat or into civilian society who were suffering from progressive Post-Traumatic Stress Disorder and were in danger of becoming, literally, walking time bombs. One only has to look at the very recent case in which former Marine Eddie Ray Routh, who was diagnosed with PTSD, gunned down two Navy SEALS who were trying to help him cope with his mental illness by taking him out to the gun range at the Rough Creek Lodge and Resort in Glen Rose, Texas, to work through his problems. The attempt, although altruistic, went horribly wrong when Routh, who, his family said, had been babbling almost incoherently in recent days, turned his semi-automatic weapon on Chris Kyle and his friend Chad Littlefield. Routh has since been arrested and charged with capital murder by Texas law enforcement. The Routh case demonstrates that even when diagnosed, PTSD is progressive and can result in deadly violence. That's why simply dumping PTSD sufferers back into society because their claims for disability were denied is more than a simple scandal—it is an example of reckless behavior in defiance of medical standards.

In the cases of accused mass killer Staff Sergeant Robert Bales and possibly of accused killer Dr. Timothy Jorden, the goings-on at Madigan Army Hospital might have had such far-reaching effects. Both soldiers had been posted to Joint Base Lewis-McChord and passed through Madigan Army Hospital. With the revelations of arbitrarily altered psychiatric diagnoses, Madigan's special forensic unit is a scandal that will impact the lives of hundreds, if not thousands, of military veterans. Soldiers who were diagnosed with Post-Traumatic Stress Disorder by a wide spectrum of behavioral health clinicians were reevaluated, absent any new diagnosis, by forensic psychiatrists who essentially functioned in the role of insurance doctors reviewing claims from a distance. They rarely even interviewed the soldiers, documenting justification for denying soldiers' claims for disability on the grounds of combat-related Post-Traumatic Stress Disorder by dismissing initial medical diagnoses and replacing them with their own findings so as to deny claims. This was reportedly done without a consultation with the soldier's diagnosing and attending clinician to find out his/her rationale for making the diagnosis and through the use of psychological testing of questionable value by itself, absent thorough face-to-face interviewing and records review of the soldier. Ostensibly, these reevaluations with altered diagnoses were conducted to weed out malingerers seeking unjustified compensation. But the mere fact that this was touted by this forensic unit as more a cost-saving measure and not as a medical issue raised official red flags among investigators, particular Senator Patty Murray, once the news became public. Did the forensic unit altering diagnoses of other clinicians at Madigan Army Hospital unleash potentially violent and suicidal young men and women back into combat or into an unprotected and unprepared public? Did they start restocking our post-Vietnam era jails, streets, and prisons with broken men and women, mainly rural kids volunteering for service to their country in the wake of September 11th who were promised the opportunity to improve their lives by serving?

What was it like at Madigan?

It was the spring of 2008 when Dr. Joe Stevens (not his real name) received a call from a friend who had developed a telepsychiatry system for the U.S. Army's Western Region (to be based at Madigan

Army Hospital) and was starting to recruit psychiatrists to staff the new project. "Everything was on the table" at this time, he assured Dr. Stevens. That meant getting in at the ground floor of a project that Stevens knew had the finest equipment. His friend, a psychiatrist who had also retired from private practice in Seattle, always executed well. So Stevens did not have to worry about this system going live and being successful.

Dr. Stevens had been working for ten years as a "rent-a-shrink" in scores of hospitals and clinics nationally and had witnessed a lot of electronic medical records going live online, only to become more trouble for nurses and doctors than they were worth. He also had experience with federal telehealth systems to service remote regions on Native American reservations. They worked and had great potential to bring modern psychiatry to regions all over North America that were struggling with economic and health conditions more like third world nations than middle-class Americans could expect from their local clinics and hospitals. The director had left, however, and Stevens thought the system would gather dust at the hospital servicing the reservation. He was certain that his friend's state-of-the-art system—for which no corners were cut, nor dimes spared, to get the best high definition teleconferencing systems available—would, like all his friend's projects, have the unwavering support from the Pentagon. Stevens could not understand how his friend could do what he did from a small suite of offices in the Old Madigan Hospital, a literal maze of confusing hallways. But he knew if there was an opportunity to help make a modern clinical IT system work, this would be the likely site for a successful startup to set the national standard of practice for integrating telepsychiatry and the largest electronic health record ever developed—the Armed Forces Health Longitudinal Tracking Application, also known as CHCS II and AHLTA.

With minimal delay in real-time communication, all specialists know from watching global satellite interviews on the news that teleconferencing is not perfect. But the War on Terror had spread America's volunteer Army, National Guard, and active reserve personnel so thin across North America, Central Asia, the Middle East, and Africa that it was obvious that Madigan's telepsychiatry project for the United States Army's Western Region had to be the solution nobody had yet developed and built out. His friend also had some sort of special mentoring in the Army that was both high up and powerful. Most importantly, the Army's expert on PTSD and suicides was on public record for promoting its use to speed up clinical interventions to prevent debilitating, and oftentimes lethal, complications of untreated PTSD and unrecognized suicidal soldiers.

Dr. Stevens believed this system could leverage scarce psych resources in the Army and eventually be transferred to the civilian world that he knew was suffering from increasingly scarce psychiatric resources. Dr. Stevens's friend even gave him permission to make contact with neurosurgical colleagues at the University of British Columbia in order to start integrating this system into NATO through the Canadian Army. UBC's department of neurosurgery was anxious to discuss collaboration because casualties were coming into Victoria and Vancouver, British Columbia, from Afghanistan. Canadian military health care was even more strapped for global combat missions than the United States'.

Tired of traveling so much, Dr. Joe Stevens started another solo private practice and was off to a fairly good start. Now if he could just add this section of the country to the service area of Madigan telepsychiatry, Stevens was fairly certain that he could connect a local military base in Corpus Christie, Texas, into the new Army's Western Region telepsychiatry project. He could even be evaluating and consulting on patients throughout the Western Region from home during the winter to avoid the worsening wetting of Pacific Northwest winters. In fact, by May 2008, he was optimistic that he would become an integral part of building out one of the best telepsychiatry systems this country had ever seen. And maybe doing so would enable him, from wherever he was, to consult on fascinating and challenging combat psychiatry cases worldwide, armed only with a specially secured laptop computer issued to military psychiatrists for practicing off the Army electronic health record, AHLTA.

But despite the optimism of a new telepsychiatric system at Madigan, things had changed, in part because the entire American economy was in a state of collapse. In so doing, the changes in government medical resource availability diminished, taking the promise of a national model for modern healthcare delivery via telepsychiatry and teleneurology with it, along with President Bush's anticipation that AHLTA would be the model for hauling civilian healthcare into the new millennium. With that squeeze on funding for military and veterans' benefits came the establishment of an ad hoc psychiatric unit at Madigan Army Medical Center that took it upon itself to act as a claims adjuster, reassessing diagnoses of long-term, mental health disabilities diagnosed by many other clinicians at Madiagan Army Medical Center. This is the story of what happened at Madigan, and it is not a pretty story. It would be a challenge to build this digital/medical bridge, but Dr. Stevens saw the opportunity to have the best of both worlds. It was the spring of 2008.

As he prepared for his interviews the next day, Dr. Stevens felt comfortable being back on a military base, again awash in memories of another war; another deployment over forty years earlier. He had been drafted out of his internship to serve in Vietnam as a newly minted physician. It had been decades since he walked the tarmac of McChord Air Force Base. It had been a lot shorter time since he had testified in an insanity trial of a murderer at a Fort Lewis Court Martial that resulted in the death penalty. That was in 1986. Now he was back.

Dr. Stevens waited in the lobby of a small hotel in Dupont, a small town off-base to the south of Fort Lewis. This is an enormous military complex, and his next meeting at Madigan Army Medical

Center would be several miles to the north up I-5. The north boundary of the recently integrated McChord AFB was another several miles. JBLM encompasses fifteen square miles and includes the major airlift capacity for rapid deployment of our forces globally and one of the major military medical facilities for both treatment and research internationally. A 500-square-mile firing range is just a few hours east over the Cascade mountains. Joint Base Lewis-McChord is one of the largest and most important military complexes within the Department of Defense portfolios, known as the primary "Power Projection Platform" west of the Rockies.

To emphasize the importance of the base, one could see that there were no other Americans in the lobby early Monday morning. There were a dozen Australian soldiers in combat fatigues waiting to be picked up for training. They were Special Forces, because Fort Lewis is home to the first Special Forces unit, to which Staff Sergeant Robert Bales was assigned. And it is home to the Madigan Army Medical Center, one of the largest military hospitals on the West Coast and one of three designated trauma centers in United States Army Medical Department (AMEDD). It has one of the largest uniformed staff of military psychiatrists outside of Walter Reed.

All graduates of the Uniformed Armed Forces School of Medicine at Walter Reed in Washington, D.C., and all veterans of recent and long deployments in Iraq were the Army's own uniformed doctors posted there. Significantly, there were four colonels and only one major among them. In addition to Dr. Stevens's friend, who did special healthcare project development for the Pentagon, there were at least six other civilian psychiatrists, most of them full-time civil service with military experience. A couple psychiatric positions were temporary slots, staffed by contract firms working nationally. There was a large inpatient unit manned by a "Colonel John," who had recently commanded the entire psychiatric services deployment for *Operation Iraqi Freedom.* He was the idealized prototype from the book *With Scalpel and Sword* and presumably career army, a likely candidate to one day become a top leader of army psychiatry like Colonel Elspeth Ritchie, Army expert on Suicides; and General Laurie Sutton, director of the Department of Defense Center of Excellence for PTSD and Traumatic Brain Injuries—both of whom have long since retired.

These were heady times for military psychiatry. Colonel John had a full-time civilian colleague. They were both off on weekends, nights and holidays. Most base psychiatrists, including Colonel John—the commanding officer of psychiatry—and civilian and military psychiatrists, rotated in managing the inpatient unit and emergency consultations throughout the hospital and ER. Suffice it to say, Joint Base is no stepping stone to Alaska, as the tradition of Seattle/Tacoma has been—but rather to Washington, D.C., for the loyal and respected few. Likewise, Madigan Army Medical Center is a flagship hospital and clinic complex for the Army, and it services all military personnel in the continental Pacific Northwest, including a fleet to the north in Everett, naval shipyards across Puget Sound in Bremerton, and the nuclear submarine base on Hood Canal. Additionally, the North Pacific Coast Guard depends on it for the care of serious illnesses, since the public health hospital in Seattle was converted to civilian use. Every commander in the United States military knows Joint Base Lewis-McChord, and few have never set foot on it or passed through it if Army docs very long.

Dr. Stevens's friend showed up, and they caught up on local news. Psychiatric communities tend to be small and close. There are few psychiatrists who were in training with them at the University of Washington whom they did not mutually know. The same was true for the community of psychiatrists trained at the Uniformed Armed Forces School of Medicine at Walter Reed Army Medical Center in Washington, D.C. They all obviously knew each other and had special ties, as would be expected from their unique training, service obligations, and combat psychiatry deployments to Iraq. They were trained in both *scalpel and sword*, too unique a breed not to be fraternal. Deployed to the combat theater, unlike the unarmed psychiatrists in Saigon during the Vietnam War, they were never without their weapons (which they knew how to use), and on occasion, they had their fingers on the triggers in Iraq. They were all well-trained and very competent doctors, but they were also soldiers who knew how to defend themselves, and would on occasion discuss their varied tours in Iraq. That was too occasional for Dr. Stevens because their narratives were all different, having served in different areas of the theater at different times and different places. So their narratives, sparse as they were, did provide a mosaic of duty and life in the Sandbox, as Iraq was known at Madigan. Although it might seem paradoxical that Army medical staff members would prefer to be in a theater of war rather than safe and secure at an Army hospital, a surprising number of staff members preferred the Iraq "Sandbox" to serving at Madigan just because service in Iraq was all about practicing medicine. Serving at Madigan was too much about playing politics and screwing around with a clunker of the computer technology called AHLTA, the military's electronic medical records system, that everyone hated. This computer database system was so flawed that it became one of the main reasons for army clinicians deciding not to re-up for additional tours. They would rather return to community service or "RTCS" than stay chained to a flawed medical records system that simply didn't work and made their jobs harder.

The subject quickly turned to business. Madigan Army Medical Center had taken delivery of millions of dollars in the finest video conferencing equipment, which was in the process of being rolled out from the furthest reaches of the Aleutian Islands in the Arctic Ocean to southern California. Indeed, everything was still on the table: Expansion throughout the western states, including Hawaii and Texas; integration with Canadian military medicine and civilian specialty support; and collaboration with neurologists and neurosurgeons at the nearby University of British Columbia in

Vancouver. There was potential for contract psychiatrists to work remotely from their homes, and there was a pool of old colleagues from the University of Washington from which to recruit for evaluation and consultation with medics face-to-face on the ground with soldiers who could be anywhere on the planet.

The prospects for this telepsychiatry project were exciting. What had been discussed by phone was really happening here on base. But there was one obstacle. Dr. Stevens would have to take time off from his private practice in Corpus Christi to learn modern Army medicine before being capable of working on his own with a secure laptop computer performing telepsychiatry to anywhere in the world from, hypothetically, anywhere in the world. This would be a sacrifice, but one worth taking to learn the clinical IT system that President Bush envisioned as a solution to many of the problems of fragmented medical care in the civilian world. Stevens had reason to believe that this would be his best chance to integrate clinical decision support of triaging into a highly sophisticated clinical IT platform that included telemedicine from numerous specialties, including telepsychiatry and teleneurology, as well as the first electronic health records covering an entire population, all army personnel, for any clinical encounter, and anywhere on earth. Was this not the opportunity of a lifetime? So Dr. Stevens would head several miles up I-5 to meet with the commander of Madigan's psychiatric department, Colonel Dave.

Dr. Stevens and Colonel Dave met in the colonel's office in the behavioral science department, a large clinic taking up a ground-level corner of the new Madigan building. It was divided between psychiatry and psychology, but Colonel Dave had overall command responsibility. This was no off-beat clinic invisible to the radar screens of AMEDD in Washington, D.C. It was important, housing about fifty offices for therapists treating soldiers and psychiatrists working with nurse practitioners, prescribing psychotropic medications for soldiers, military dependents, and retired military, too. Colonel

Dave, happy to be back from Iraq, was a child psychiatrist and a low-profile kind of commander—and not very intimidating in his combat fatigues and black beret. Nobody was visibly armed in the clinic. Like Stevens's friend, Colonel Dave was working on projects for the Pentagon, mainly having to do with the fascinating new problems of the all-volunteer Army that involved multiple deployments and husband-and-wife active-duty couples rarely being deployed at same time.

The Surgeon General of the Army was particularly interested in the unique stresses of multiple deployments, oftentimes of both parents, on children. He had developed special books for parents and children to read in preparation for deployment. Stevens did not know at the time, however, that he would actually come to depend on them for supporting deployment of experienced NCOs who had been deployed so much that their families were suffering. This was a special war with special skills needed, but not every soldier could fill the needs. So some were overworked in support of the mission. Nowhere was this truer than with experienced NCOs who had proven from experience that they could recognize the suspicious signs of an IED up ahead, or the guy who could defuse it. Some families suffered more than others, including those with mothers who had to deploy to dangerous assignments, even though they were not infantry. Transport and logistics in the War on Terror is very dangerous, and women drove a lot of trucks through a lot of treacherous real estate.

Dr. Stevens and Colonel Dave came from different generations, but neither from the greatest one that had won World War II. It went without saying, therefore, that the wars in Iraq and Afghanistan, like Vietnam, were dirty little wars. There was no gung-ho; just realities of this nation's response to the attacks of September 11th. Cheney said it would take a long time, but in May 2008, who at Madigan would have a clue what he meant when he made that prediction?

The meeting with Colonel Dave went well enough that Stevens felt confident he could start practicing on the psychiatric—or prescribing—side of the behavioral health clinic and pull the routine emergency call as he had in numerous hospitals from coast to coast. The military ER could not be that different, he thought.

As they left the office, saying nice things about getting together again and exchanging professional cards, a stout colonel in combat fatigues approached the office with obvious urgency. He seemed a bit intrusive, but obviously had what Stevens thought to be a serious problem that needed the attention of his commander. Colonel Dave introduced the two psychiatrists, and they hastily shook hands in indifferent politeness. This man seemed too frustrated and preoccupied for any small talk. It was a bit odd that he unloaded right in front of a perfect stranger, but perhaps he knew the civilian was a psychiatrist, too, and likely to come on board. Then he unloaded as if he was in private office with Commander Dave: "This guy's case is a mess. We got to get something done about these problems. They're too many of them."

This was Colonel William Keppler, later to be caught up in a scandal for running a forensic unit at Madigan that reviewed other clinicians' diagnoses, and rarely, if ever, consulted with these other clinicians—they simply changed many of the original diagnoses, denying these soldiers disability benefits after discharge. Reportedly, some of these reviews included forensic psychiatric interviews, and presumably in all cases, administration of an MMPI test. Colonel Keppler never demonstrated any bravado and frequently referenced his disgust with the military medical system, asserting that the system was broken and that he was returning to civilian service. This was an obvious reference to his dissatisfaction with the military healthcare system, and as it became more clear, its medical disability system.

Joint Base Lewis-McChord is an enormous campus with numerous isolated, off-beat buildings housing clinics such as the telepsychiatry development office, the Traumatic Brain Injury

Clinic, the disability doctors reviewing medical evaluation boards for medical discharges from the army, and the McChord Air Force Base Clinic. But the Madigan Army Medical Center is the obvious central hub for everything, including the general who commands the hospital and a beautiful reflecting pond with a geyser for a fountain. There are plenty of geese to keep misbehaving soldiers busy scraping up their excrement from the sidewalks, a modern arcade with signs designating various specialty clinics, and a bright, busy enclosed plaza with comfortable seating for patients and families. All of this might remind one of a relaxed resort—except for an occasional soldier with a circumferential scar cutting through his forehead who would remind one that this is not a high-end suburban hospital, but an army hospital responsible for the care of some of the most critically wounded and critically important warriors for the War on Terror. It would never have been built after the events of September 11th. It was obviously for another era that would appeal to soldiers seeking a good career and maintaining readiness for rapid projection of power globally. Certainly it was not built as a military hospital for a nation that had been attacked and remained vulnerable to more attacks. In fact, the spread-out layout of the old hospital, rather than a large multi-story facility, was more the result of the U.S. fear at the outset of World War II that the Northwest would be bombed by the Japanese.

The behavioral health clinic where Colonel Dave was interviewing a civilian candidate occupied the entire northwest corner of the building. The forensic unit was far removed from it. However, that unit was close enough that Colonel Keppler was in regular communication regarding patients with all the psychiatrists in the hospital and behavioral health clinic. Having heard what he had been doing in his office, it came as a surprise to Dr. Stevens that Keppler's office was not at all closed to doctors needing to talk with him about various issues. Colonel Keppler pretty much steered clear of evaluating primary psychiatric disabilities that had no medical surgical injuries. His reported duty was to do the less controversial "secondaries," where a medical/surgical specialist had already determined disability. Keppler only had to determine associated—or comorbid—psychiatric impairment resulting from medical-surgical disability. This was not such a contentious issue in the obviously head-injured soldiers with those surgical scars appearing like unholy halos, or serious burn cases and amputees. He was so open with colleagues about his frustration with the psychiatric disability system—particularly for soldiers medically discharged after having been caught abusing illegal drugs—that it is unlikely that nobody else in the army chain of command knew that he did more in his forensic office than evaluate forensic cases for comorbid and associated psychiatric complications of physical wounds, competency to stand trial, or insanity defenses. As news stories revealed in 2012, we recently learned just how much more when the story of the scandal broke out in the headlines.

According to the *Seattle Times* in an article on June 10, 2012, an Army doctor at Madigan was suspended over his comments regarding PTSD. The article revealed that two Madigan Army psychiatrists were removed from their duties in the clinic because of allegations that PTSD diagnoses of soldiers had been mishandled when diagnoses of soldiers with PTSD were reversed. Specifically, the article said, "A Madigan Army Medical Center psychiatrist who screens soldiers for PTSD has been removed from clinical duties while investigators look into controversial remarks he made about patients and the financial costs of disability benefits, according to U.S. Sen. Patty Murray." That doctor was William Keppler, who had retired, but who led a forensic psychiatric team in charge of reevaluating PTSD in soldiers for whom medical boards were ordered for their ultimate medical retirement at Joint Base Lewis-McChord. Indeed, many millions of dollars in lifetime benefits were at stake that could not be reversed once stamped with final approval for medical discharge. Because of Keppler's statements that threw into question his role in assessing PTSD disability claims, the Army began a complete review of the work of that forensic unit.

On February 8, 2013, the *Seattle Times* reported that Dr. Russel Hicks, a fifteen-year member of the medical staff, was suspended from Madigan Army Medical Center, where he was a psychiatrist. Although the claims against him were related to "alleged problems with patient care," according to the report, Dr. Hicks told the paper he thought the suspension was a retaliatory act because of information he supplied to the Army investigators reviewing the hospital's PTSD diagnosis program.

Scope and Nature of the Problem at Madigan

According to the Army Surgeon General Patricia Horoho, who has since testified before Senator Patty Murray's subcommittee, the problem is embedded in the anomalous role of forensic psychiatry at Madigan and across the military healthcare landscape. General Horoho told Senator Murray, by way of assurances, that she was investigating whether the problems at Madigan were systemic: whether there were reversals of psychiatric diagnoses of PTSD across the military hospital system, or if they were localized at Madigan. They were looking, Horoho said, for "variants across the processes." She explained that forensic psychiatry introduces "variance into the integrated disability evaluation system process." Were these variants fair or unfair in treating service members? This is the question the Army Surgeon General is asking, and what her investigation, she promised Senator Murray, will determine. Was what happened at Lewis-McChord a local problem, or a problem across the entire system? Senator Murray and the Army both want that answer.

We wonder, however, what General Horoho meant by "variants across its processes?" And what is the integrated disability evaluation system process of the Army? And what should we understand in her conclusion that "an inspector general investigation will look at variants or systemic issues across Army medicine," as if General Horoho suspected the problem might not be isolated to Magidan?

This statement could be euphemistically misleading inasmuch as it implies that the Army simply plans to walk away from the problem once they assure the Senate committee that whatever the problem was at Madigan, they've got the problem covered. Her assurance to the committee that it was her responsibility to "make sure that we were fairly treating our service members and providing them the best care possible" it was a bureaucratic way of sweeping away the problem because it never addressed the issue, which was that legitimate medical diagnoses were summarily reversed by a board of claims adjusters with medical degrees who suspected that those diagnosed with a mental illness were defrauding the military. General Horoho, without dealing with the medical and ethical specifics of the problem, made a promise that the Army would investigate, and that they would get back to Senator Murray with answers. Who could possibly disagree with her on that, except those wanting to know upon what medical basis the forensic psychiatric team made its decisions?

The Army did indeed conduct a cursory investigation, lasting a little over a month, and said they determined that the problem of reversing diagnoses of PTSD was not systemic; it was localized at Madigan. According to the Army Vice Chief of Staff, General Lloyd Austin, the forensic psychiatric test used at Madigan will no longer be used because what was used for civilian psychiatric evaluations was not "optimal" for military evaluations. Here's the difference, at least for our purposes. A forensic evaluation is adversarial, designed to ferret out dissemblers or malingerers. It is based on challenging a claim so as to verify its legitimacy. It is almost as if the evaluator for the Army becomes a claims adjuster validating a claim by a soldier seeking disability compensation, but doing it from an adversarial perspective. The focus is on challenging a diagnosis. For military purposes, the test for PTSD has to be conducted to address symptoms and assess treatment methodologies. The Army determined that forensic—designed to challenge—is not the best medical practice, and thus the forensic unit, headed up at Madigan, will not be reinstated, although the Army promised that the commander of the hospital, Colonel Dallas Homas, will be reinstated. And since forensic evaluations were only conducted by the unit at Madigan, the Army, at least by its own explanation, is off the hook.

If the Army is seeking to exonerate itself through its investigation of variances in order to whitewash and then discard what was going on in the forensic psychiatric unit at Madigan, it would be reminiscent of the governor's report concerning the mass murders at Virginia Tech, the federal commission reviewing the attacks on September 11th, and yes the Warren Commission. Blue-ribbon panels are sometimes created for the express purpose of assigning blame and isolating the government from any tort liability deriving from an incident. Thus we believe that although the military does evaluate long-term disability claims, the forensic unit at Madigan might have been an early experiment in aggressive claims adjustment because the Pentagon feared, as former Defense Secretary prophesized, that it would be turned into a long-term disability insurance company.

We compare the Army Inspector General's review of the Madigan scandal to other officially empanelled commissions, just to show how a high-profile incident like altering diagnoses at Madigan Hospital could be a "variance" peculiar to the Madigan Army Medical Center, Joint Base Lewis-McChord, and the headquarters of the Western Army Region by a rogue psychiatrist, or it could be a "variance" at other military bases. Or, it could be a variance, as the Surgeon General hinted, between the actual practice of forensic psychiatry throughout the military medical system, specifically some forensic psychiatrists specializing in reviews of disability determinations within "the process" of the Army's "integrated disability evaluation system." It may, in the Surgeon General's euphemistic paradigm, therefore be at variance with forensic psychiatrists who do only psychiatric evaluations for court martials, such as the mass murder trials of Hasan and Bales. In other words, there are two standards: one for disability compensation, and one for plain, old-fashioned, psychiatric evaluations, including forensic psychiatric exams.

Although the Army's investigation into the Madigan Army Medical Center's forensic psychiatric unit and their arbitrary altering of diagnoses made by a spectrum of clinicians at Madigan has been ostensibly completed, there has been no response to a letter from the founder of the Seattle Forensic Institute questioning why medical disciplinary, or even criminal charges, have not been brought against this forensic unit: a cabal of military compensation evaluators who methodically corrupted the system, as it was revealed in the Senate hearings and in the *Seattle Times*, by deliberately altering psychiatric evaluations of PTSD to deny disability compensation claims. In so doing, this forensic unit unleashed mentally ill and potentially dangerous, ticking time bombs upon other soldiers in their unit, civilian populations in theaters of war, and upon the American public and its public safety and health networks. Too much time has elapsed for such a response, and the state of Washington does have a strong interest in this matter, as do the doctors involved, who are civilians presumably licensed by the state of Washington.

The scandal at Madigan reached the desk of Washington Senator Patty Murray when the ombudsman at Madigan went to her with the story of how medical records were altered to deny disability compensation to veterans for the ostensible reason of saving taxpayer dollars. The Pentagon was unhappy with that type of whistle-blowing, but once the secret was out, it took on a life of its own. However, the Army pushed back, saying that its Army Auditing Agency was now investigating the ombudsman for his role in possibly costing the government over $1.5 million per soldier denied disability claims as the result of actions taken by the Madigan forensic psychiatric unit. Army officers argue that the ombudsman had no business going to Senator Murray because the ombudsman's job is to work within the Army chain of command, not outside the chain of command. A veteran psychiatrist without prior problems at Madigan who also blew the whistle on this forensic unit has now been suspended for "other issues," coincidentally never observed before in many years of practice at Madigan.

Thus, following what appears to be Army logic, what happens in the United States Army may not be anyone else's business because of its ingrown general staff officer culture. We are supposed to trust without question the Army's internal investigation while the ombudsman becomes a matter of investigation and implied punishment for blowing the whistle to Congress. But what is the Army's complaint; disclosure of a truth? Is the alteration of diagnoses, seemingly conducted very arbitrarily without consulting the diagnosing physician, a legal or ethical act? We suggest that, Army chain of command notwithstanding, the soldiers (both active duty and veterans), families of soldiers, and military and contract civilian clinicians are collectively subject to and protected by the rights of the rule of law, particularly if clinicians stand to incur liability if a combat vet with PTSD commits a heinous crime due to mental illness—a mental illness that was diagnosed but not treated because the Army forced the clinician to change the veteran's medical records so as to deny him or her disability compensation. Looking at Adam Lanza's Sandy Hook shootings and Aurora shooter James Holmes's University of Colorado models, what the Army did at Madigan could similarly be a disaster in the making because of either underdiagnosing, undertreating, or both.

Considering the case of Staff Sergeant Robert Bales: If the Army knew that Bales was suffering from PTSD, and yet deployed him because his real problems were covered up at Madigan in the organized manipulation of military personnel medical records, the Army could not only be violating its own rules of engagement—which must align with international law, as well as with medical ethics and good old American morality—but also actually breaking the law under the

Code of Military Justice with its falsification of military records. It is a scandal of potentially great magnitude, because not only are Army personnel involved, but presumably also civilian psychiatrists working within one hour of the capital of Washington State and its Board of Medical Licensing in Olympia. It is unlikely that any psychiatrist really knows whether his diagnoses were, in fact, being reviewed by this forensic unit, even though they likely worked side-by-side with these same psychiatrists in sharing emergency psychiatric call at nights, on weekends and during holidays! Hardly the making of good faith and trust on the front lines of military medicine.

Senator Patty Murray gently, but nevertheless relentlessly, questioned General Horoho at hearings into the Madigan scandal. Why was Senator Murray selected to take this to the United States public? Because she happened to be close by when the Army's ombudsman decided to go outside? Or was it because she represented the state of Washington? These soldiers were legal residents of the state of Washington during their time at Fort Lewis and Madigan, whether living on base or off. The alleged leader of this rogue forensic unit was a retired military psychiatrist, presumably—although not absolutely necessarily—licensed in the state of Washington. It is the opinion of the authors that basic rules of law apply in this case, and that it is not simply a matter for internal investigation. In fact, should the commander of Madigan Hospital during peak years of these goings-on be present herself as totally objective and without knowledge of these events during her watch, there may be an issue of vicarious liability. Vicarious liability, a term out of tort law, might attach even if it was possible that she was totally blind to the goings-on, because for two years she worked under the same roof as members of this allegedly rogue unit, was the boss of the entire command, and likely had frequent encounters with the doctors involved. Is she objective enough, therefore, to conduct an investigation that could possibly inculpate her? Should she not also remove herself from any role in this investigation because she could very possibly be party to it, or even an integral part of the operation? The Army has to remove the slightest appearance of a self-serving cover-up.

Scope of Problem to Date

During Senator Murray's committee hearing on the reportedly "inappropriate" outspoken comments by the leader of the forensic unit at Madigan and his unit's arbitrary reversal of diagnoses of PTSD in returning combat veterans in an adversarial claims investigation, a muted and polite exchange between Senator Murray, Secretary of the Army McHugh, Surgeon General Horoho, and General Odierha seemed to calm the waters publicly. Senator Murray conveyed her sense of discouragement, having had to return to DOD heads with more disturbing news. Many soldiers, for all intents and purposes, are getting screwed over—the only way to put it—by the military when seeking help for "invisible wounds of war," specifically emotional distress, severe sleep problems, wafer-thin resiliency in the face of everyday challenges, flashbacks of horrors of combat, and avoidant behaviors damaging to personal lives, all as a result of saving their lives and the lives of others in combat zones. Although the problem is shocking in both the individual hubris of doctors on this forensic team and the numbers of patients rescreened, as well as the number of diagnoses arbitrarily reversed, the calming reassurance from the Army brass in response to repeated questions was alarming for its very soothing tone, which was not prosecutorial enough in light of the serious circumstances and potentially deadly consequences. It is what one might refer to politely as cognitive dissonance. Where is the outrage? Where is the moral indignation of Senator Murray, demanding to know why a unit at Madigan declared itself to be the Army's insurance claims adjusters looking for reasons to deny disability to sick veterans?

That one Army psychiatrist (with a partner or two in a single hospital) could be doing this type of official medical records manipulation of his own accord since on active duty in 2007 and into retirement, continuing it as a contract civil service doctor at the same hospital well into 2012, suggests that there was an administrative cover-up in place. Where it started, how it was communicated, the extent of those involved, and how high up it went are all matters to be investigated. However, internal investigations notwithstanding, because Sergeant Bales came from this base and was allegedly screened and declared fit for duty before committing the atrocities in Afghanistan—and because the inappropriateness of this forensic unit was reported by the *Seattle Times* almost concurrently—the question, of course, naturally arose: Could his atrocities be laid on the doorstep of this Madigan forensic unit? Was Bales one whose diagnosis had been reversed at Madigan, and then deployed from Joint Base Lewis-McChord with no psych problems? Or, if he was not subject to the unit, did the spillover effects from this unit's power and influence at Madigan, as in the associated closure of Madigan's specialized PTSD clinic, create a climate of diagnostic nihilism among clinicians? Or, worse yet, was there a literal meltdown of clinical services for pre-deployment fitness-for-duty examinations, so that Bales's "S" profile for psychiatric status was simply neglected?

The forensic unit, if so justified for its existence at Madigan, should be the watchdog for fitness-for-duty profiles to make certain that mentally deranged—or at-risk soldiers, like Robert Bales—were not being deployed back into sensitive and brittle combat situations against their vocal objections. If there is justification for such a unit like this, it is for that purpose. But where were the eyes of this unit when Bales vocally objected to a fourth deployment where he, more than apparently anyone else, knew he was not fit for the duties because of his combat injuries? It is not necessarily the direct association between this unit and the Bales case, but rather the indirect one— one of diversion of critical resources, namely scarce Army psychiatric resources, to a work scope more the domain of claims adjudication at Department of Veterans Affairs, rather than combat psychiatry. This allegedly rogue operation at Madigan started while its leader was on active duty as a combat psychiatrist, not an insurance doctor working for Department of Veterans Affairs.

Bales's attorney says he was not neglected, nor had his records been altered, because he had not been diagnosed with PTSD and sent for a medical evaluation board—the apparent triggering event that was the signal for Colonel Keppler to review the medical records for consideration of reversing diagnoses or even eliminating diagnoses. Was he evaluated for PTSD? Was PTSD, or any of its diagnostic criteria—such as nightmares requiring treatment with Prazosin—ever entered into AHLTA as one or some of his problems? It must be remembered that 1,680 patients were allegedly screened by Keppler's unit, more than 690 of whom had been diagnosed with Post-Traumatic Stress Disorder, according to Senator Murray. The psychiatric team reversed more than 290 of those diagnoses, or about 40 percent. That is a huge number of altered diagnoses, regardless of the medical institution in which it is occurring. During the hearing, there was no acknowledgement that this process was wrong in any way, hence the absence of official outrage. But the Senator was repeatedly assured that the matter was being investigated, both for its standard of service—a standard unheard of—and for evidence that it was systemic, rather than simply the actions of a rogue psychiatrist both outspoken on the need to cut the costs of psychiatric disability and operating quite visibly at Madigan since 2007. What happened to the command structure at Madigan, and why weren't any medical summary reports submitted up the chain of command? Where was General Horoho while this was going on within her visual fields? These military medical officers would naturally share the same water cooler on occasion, simply because the architecture of Madigan Army Medical Center provided places for staff to congregate. They certainly were not absolute total strangers.

"To this point, we don't see any evidence of this being systemic," Secretary of the Army McHugh testified to Senator Murray's committee. "But as you and I have discussed," he said, referring to Murray, "We want to make sure that where this was inappropriate, it was an isolated case, and if it were not, to make sure we address it as holistically as we're trying to address it at Madigan." In other words, the secretary was assuring the Senate that the Army wanted to make sure that Colonel Keppler and his unit was like the character Kurtz in Conrad's *Heart of Darkness* and Coppola's *Apocalypse Now*: a single rogue official, who carved out his own mini command and ran it his own way. However, given the way today's Army works, and the way the medical profession operates, the secretary's assurances make no sense whatsoever. In other words, we simply don't buy it. Something stinks at the very top.

Army Chief of Staff, General Odierno, was at the secretary's side, reassuring Senator Murray that the soldiers' good health and best care was the primary mission of Army medicine. If there could be no disagreement with Odierno's statement in principle, why was this an issue in the first place, an issue going all the way up across every desk top in the military command until floating right past the Army Chief of Staff, and landing in the office of the Secretary of the Army? What could have gone wrong? Even if Senator Murray, the Army Surgeon General, the Army Chief of Staff, and the Secretary of the Army all agree, the questions linger because American taxpayers, despite the rabid fanaticism over budget deficits, nevertheless do not want medical decisions made for our troops based on financial concerns. There are other ways to save money that don't involve compromising the lives of combat troops and veterans, and quite possibly, public safety and health officers, as well as innocent civilians.

Senator Murray said that the United States Congress, and not Colonel Keppler, makes the decision about how to pay for the care of soldiers. So how could any doctor—a single psychiatrist—bestow upon himself a power that would be the cause of felony charges and loss of licensure in a civilian clinical environment? That is the question both General Horoho and Secretary McHugh promised to answer, and which they have answered by removing the forensic psychiatric unit from Madigan. They claimed no knowledge of Colonel Keppler's activities, but are isolating the problem. However, they gave the unit a very wide berth with such statements as "Doctors having different opinions on different patients," natural disagreements among clinicians, standards of practice throughout the system that should not allow for such extreme deviations from the curve, and other explanations. But they did not address what Keppler was saying about changing medical diagnoses to deny disability claims, other than to say that was not their point of view on the purpose of medical evaluations. Certainly cost should not be a factor, they all agreed.

According to Army reports, "Madigan psychiatrists used objective testing to determine which soldiers had 'significant mental illness that was compensable.' One of those tests the Madigan forensic team used is called the Minnesota Multiphasic Personality Inventory (MMPI). In one patient file reviewed by the *Seattle Times*, a forensic-team member said the validity of the MMPI has been confirmed by multiple studies and has 'shown the best resolution' in separating 'PTSD simulators from actual patients.'"

Unfortunately, the validity of the MMPI for discriminating between PTSD and malingering is highly controversial, particularly if it is the central validating tool that is used without face-to-face interviews and complementary tests now available. And what MMPI was used? The test was found to be invalid on a stand-alone basis for the diagnosis of PTSD in screening both incest victims and Vietnam vets after the inclusion of Post-Traumatic Stress Disorder in the Diagnostic Statistical Manual in 1980. An attempt to find a better MMPI was made with the Mississippi MMPI version for PTSD, but that was not valid on a stand-alone basis either. In fact, the MMPI is very misleading in psychiatric diagnostics in the wake of extreme trauma, largely because the questions addressed by the subject cannot filter out and distinguish feelings of unreality that show high peaks on psychoticism in non-psychotic patients. And such peaks can be misinterpreted, even parsed by computerized scoring as exaggeration; thus the deliberate manipulation of a malingerer.

How did this unit differentiate the MMPI that truly was that of exaggeration by a malingerer from that of a soldier who simply subscribed to questions originally calibrated half a century ago for psychosis when the soldier feels like he's going crazy? That is a real problem every clinician working with this population is aware of. The MMPI, and certain modernized versions of it, can be helpful tools, but they are not, by themselves, capable of reliably or validly discriminating PTSD from malingering or other psychiatric disorders—certainly not at the level of certainty required for such critical determinations made for military fitness-for-duty examinations. Is that not what these really were, or what they were replacing?

The validity scales are therefore often affected by the exaggeration of feelings, rather than a deliberate intent to control diagnostics. But that exaggeration—as the forensic unit presupposed to be common across all populations, including PTSD—simply is not the silver bullet for diagnosing malingering. Much more needs to be done to distinguish the reportedly 1 percent malingerering VA claimants seeking disability from the compensation-seeking real patient and the truly disabled combat vet. Projective testing and sleep lab studies are of value, but there is no alternative for unbiased, empathic and objective face-to-face interviews with returning soldiers, along with careful study of their combat histories. That can be done, and it is the standard of practice for military fitness-for-duty examinations. Was that done? Sadly, such broad spectrum and in-depth psychiatric and psychological diagnostics was likely never done with so many cases in such a high-volume clinic where the PTSD clinic was, reportedly for other reasons, being closed.

As a postscript to the investigation into Madigan, the Army admits to the inadequacy of the MMPI (Minnesota Multiphasic

Personality Inventory) and has since discontinued its use, as well as discontinuing the forensic psychiatric unit at Madigan. But we predict there will still be more fallout from this scandal.

As the shrill sound of the whistle-blower fades away, those involved with the Army medical system, particularly at Madigan, are left to wonder whether there is an undiagnosed epidemic of PTSD among troops that were rotated through Joint Base Lewis-McChord, and whether the carriers of that PTSD pathogen are at risk for dangerousness and violence to themselves and others? We should not have to wait to discover the results in morning newspaper headlines or on the evening news.

Chapter 9

Active Duty Suicides in the Military: Causalities and Approaches to Treatment

As of 2010, U.S. military suicides average over twenty per day.

This week's edition of *Time* magazine reported that the U.S. Representative from Washington State, Jim McDermott, speaking to fellow House members, describes military suicides as an "epidemic." "I would like to take $10 million out of a $5 billion fund in this amendment to go beyond the funding for existing suicide prevention services, and toward modifying the culture that keeps some from seeking help," he has advocated, noting that whatever progress is made in suicide prevention will only be "fleeting" unless the Army, and the country at large, reduces the "stigma" that attaches when an active-duty service person seeks psychological health services. If seeking such services jeopardizes a soldier's career, the Pentagon is doing a disservice to its combat personnel, Representative McDermott argued.

"McDermott said that it was easy enough to send our young men and women off to war, but he asked, 'What do we do when the people come home? We forget them.'" There is a false assumption among people in government and among the public at large that people returning from combat should have the wherewithal to straighten themselves out and simply return to their former lives. However, many returning vets cannot slip back into their former lives without some form of help or psychological counseling. Absent help, those who are suffering from mental illness could become desperate and hopeless and ultimately look to suicide as a relief. "That shouldn't happen to a twenty-four-year-old kid, man or woman, who has been in Afghanistan," Representative McDermott said.

As if to underscore the point, a recent article in the *New York Times* also cited a number of sources, including former Secretary of Defense Robert Gates, as saying that the suicide rate in the army was out of control and growing. Similar frustration expressed from Capitol Hill by Congressman McDermott is echoed by current Secretary of Defense, Leon Panetta, who calls the epidemic of suicides among U.S. soldiers the most frustrating problem he faces. Ironically, as the war winds down, promising fewer if any deployments to the combat zone, the suicide rate is spiking upwards. Army suicide expert, Colonel Elspeth Ritchie, M.D., calls this spike a lagging indicator, as the Army's suicide rate grows larger than the age-adjusted civilian rate of suicide.

And it can go on for years, as this country tries to assimilate nearly three million combat veterans from the War on Terror into society safely and with the dignity they deserve. So far, homicide rates, felony assaults, and criminal incarcerations are not promising. Nor is there much hope being offered at the level of the United States Cabinet, other than rhetoric in support of our heroes.

If documented reports of completed suicides and Dr. Ritchie's explanation for their rise is correct, years of the daily costs in human life for this War on Terror lie ahead. Similar to Vietnam, a whole generation threatens to be deeply wounded. "U.S. Military Suicides in first 155 Days of 2012 = 154 Dead," wrote Mark Thompson in *Time* magazine on June 12, 2012. That is more than this year's killed in action (KIA) rate in Operation Enduring Freedom (OEF), the technical term for the War on Terror now that *Operation Iraqi Freedom* (OIF) is officially over.

The National Institute of Mental Health completed an initial epidemiological study of Army suicides, "Study to Assess Risk and Resilience in Service-Members" (STARRS), and submitted its initial findings to the Secretary of Health in the Department of Defense in May 2011. Although the results were eye-opening to Pentagon officials more than one year ago, it is even more sobering now, because more soldiers took their own lives in the first half of 2012 as killed themselves in all of 2011. Documented completed suicides in the military reached 154 in just the first 155 days of 2012, compared with 130 over the same period in 2011. From critiques of military suicides following combat in Vietnam, we know that documented completed suicides are likely conservative due to underreporting.

It is even more staggering to hear in wartime that 50 percent more troops killed themselves than were killed in action in Afghanistan this year. The military has traditionally had a lower age-adjusted rate of completed suicides than its civilian peer population, but now it has the highest suicide toll since it has been reliably tracked in the U.S. military, at least since September 11th.

The Army "Study to Assess Risk and Resilience in Service-Members" (STARRS) examined the records of nearly one million soldiers who served in Iraq or Afghanistan between 2004 and 2008. Unfortunately, the National Guard and active reserves were left out. That glaring gap in population selection will be a serious flaw in the research due to the disproportionate burden both the Guard and reservists have had in the War on Terror. That burden has not only been disproportionate in terms of deployments relative to expected duration of service, but in its unique stress on families integrated into civilian communities, rather than military communities better capable of providing support for dependents during deployment. There is no official explanation for sending the National Guard to Afghanistan now. It might be reasonably questioned if there ever was one in the first place, with, perhaps, the exception of immediate post-September 11th months, because of total lack of military preparedness in our all-volunteer army and presidential failure to institute emergency conscription.

But for nearly one million active-duty volunteer soldiers studied in that four-year time-span, 389 completed suicides were documented. In this four-year time period, the suicide rate doubled from an average of about 100 per year to 400 per year in 2012. The striking spike of completed suicides in deployed females, although numerically small in number and at a lower rate than males, raises serious questions about circumstances surrounding their deaths, specifically in the face of only-recently published reports of sexual assaults in the military. Race appeared to be a factor also, but specifics are probably too scattered to be meaningful. Interestingly though the study did not distinguish between South Asians and East Asians. One would wonder what the rate is for Pakistani-American troops, but Pakistanis are curiously grouped with Korean and Japanese-Americans in this study. Marriage appears to be a protective factor of about two to one, but there are no demographic details that might explain this finding. Researchers stated that the Army does not distinguish between married and unmarried soldiers in terms of types or numbers of deployments.

Risk factors studied in STARRS were designed to inform the army for purposes of actionable force health protection measures to be taken. They included the following:

1. Age
2. Sex
3. Religion (more and more frequently, "none")—Strong, conservative religious values are a protective factor against suicide.

4. Education
5. Rank
6. Promotions
7. Stop-loss status for soldiers held beyond contractual terms of enlistment, because they cannot be replaced in combat theater.
8. Duration of military service.

The following risk factors still need to be studied and reported on by ongoing STARRS research:

1. Military specialty (MOS)—i.e., transport, medic, or infantryman. Unless this research is done with measures that trap the dynamics of shifting specialty assignments, correlations will be meaningless in regard to MOS. Specialties in this war are not static and are in turmoil because of what is known as "tempo." "Tempo" technically means rapid shifting of forces to hot combat areas, a perfect example of which was the Surge in Iraq. Tempo, however, can also be a euphemism for what really is perceived from the ground by the troops and their commanders as strategic, political, and command failures in the Pentagon.

"The Navy also is feeling the strain," said Vice Chief of Naval Operations, Admiral Patrick Walsh, even though ground forces are doing most of the fighting. The sea service has assigned thousands of sailors to support jobs ashore in the Middle East, using them to fill jobs that normally would be done by soldiers. Walsh warned years ago that the Navy's ability to maintain ships and aircraft will be imperiled unless lawmakers soon provide billions in extra funding sought by the Army and Marines to continue operations in Iraq. Without that money, Pentagon leaders will tap Navy and other noncombat accounts to pay war bills, he suggested. The Army is seeking an additional $66.5 billion and the Marines $1.8 billion this year for war-related expenses. How these high-level budgetary fights in the Capitol flowed down to force protection and troop morale is unknown.

2. Leadership—studies show competence of field commanders is directly proportional to resilience of troops to PTSD. A good leader is known to protect his troops and not take unnecessary risks. Why did most field lieutenants who were KIA in Vietnam die with American bullets in their backs? What actually was "fragging," and why did it occur? It occurred, most likely, because young officers were trying to get combat experience for their career records at the expense of force protection, which meant taking unnecessary risks that put their men in danger. Many paid with their lives in Vietnam, although fragging is way underreported by officials. Unless something is done about the current rear-guard action in Afghanistan, the same is going to occur, either here or in retribution back home. Soldiers who have been deployed know who these competent officers and NCOs are. There are leaders who have been deployed and motivated to return to combat in order to reduce a unit's casualties and help young men deal with death. Such commanders, whether officers or EMs, do exist in the military, and their influence on suicidality, although an opaque area in military culture, needs to be studied within the context of "Unit Assigned"—because if their influence reduced the suicide rate, it will tell us a lot about how strong leadership enhances bonding within a unit and promotes resiliency among the troops serving therein. If not, again, there will be a significant loss of meaningful correlation. It is known, for example, that units fighting in Baquba were in high intensity combat with a determined and brutal foe, one oftentimes invisible. But there were units that came in during the Surge to back them up. To designate units and associated casualty rates, it must be known that some units were already on the ground and some came in during the Surge to back them up. All need to be studied and compared to ensure meaningful correlation.

An example of how poor leadership affects the likelihood of a soldier developing PTSD is the case of Ronald Biggs, a private investigator who could not drive over the Cascade Mountains in the winter. In fact, he was homebound with agoraphobia if snow was on the ground. Every year he traveled to Germany, searching for surviving tank commanders who decimated his unit during the Battle of the Bulge.

Private Biggs was drafted late in the war, but arrived in Europe just in time for the Battle of the Bulge. He was rushed to the front in a heavy snowstorm. An open field separated his unit from a German tank emplacement that fired on them every time there was movement. Suddenly his commander, a lieutenant with a "British accent of some kind, maybe Canadian," ordered the men to charge. It was broad daylight, and the troops followed him onto the snow-white fields, their helmets and rifles barrels catching the morning sun. Easy targets, they were mowed down by withering enemy fire.

Biggs survived the machine gun rounds whizzing over his head as he hit the ground. Amidst the chaos of screaming wounded, Biggs crawled back to some brush and played possum in the snow. When night fell, he crawled to safety and was hospitalized for frostbite. He was the only survivor. After twenty trips to Germany after the war, he was able to locate most of the German tank commanders holding that field. He finally got closure when he found some who recalled the massacre and said, "Wir alles kennan das ihren Captain veruckt wahr. Wir konnte ihm nichts verstehen! Einfach—Veruckt! Alles tot ausser du!" (We all knew that your captain was crazy. We could not understand him [his actions]. Simply crazy. All dead except you.)

Ronald Biggs never told anyone in thirty years why he could not cross the Cascades in the winter and traveled to Germany so often, but he had to make closure. His commander was suicidal. Biggs had suffered PTSD because of him and had disabling survival guilt that compelled him to his obsessive search for closure.

3. Personal Weapons or Vehicles Owned—The soldier's gun is an extension of his trigger finger. When the impulse for suicide arises in a shattered mind and brain, the job gets done. Men most often kill themselves with guns, and states with the most guns per capita,

such as Arizona, do indeed have higher suicide rates than those with fewer guns per capita, such as New Jersey. Taking the active duty military as a state, one can safely assume the per capita ratio of guns per person is 100 percent. And soldiers often sleep with their guns, ready to fire in self-defense should the need arise.

4. Disciplinary problems—i.e., missing morning formation with documented panic attacks, such as the case of Thomas Stroh. Stroh, 21, who died when he drove into a head-on collision with a truck in Oregon, was about to be disciplined by the Army—confined to the barracks—for spousal abuse and being drunk on duty. It is apparent that the Army was not aware of the depth of Stroh's desperation over the collapse of his relationship until after Stroh had died and the Army collected his belongings from his house at the base. Although officials thought that Stroh's wife and child had left the house, they discovered their bodies hidden in a closet and covered in blood. Both had been shot to death. It was only then that it became apparent that Stroh had likely killed them and then took his own life, seeing no way out of his despair.

5. Failed drug tests—Marijuana used for self-medication for panic attacks and hyper-arousal found in a spot urine test can lead to disciplinary actions that can be the straw breaking a brittle back. Marijuana is still a tier-one drug, and its possession, under federal law, is a criminal offense.

6. Involvement with a criminal justice system off base, such as with a DWI, as in the case of Thomas Stroh, or assault with a deadly weapon on public safety offices, as in the case of so many soldiers at odds with the society that sent them to war with no meaningful provision for taking care of them when they returned.

7. Researchers in STARRS will also review non-suicidal deaths, presumably those involving single passenger accidents with life insurance paid to spouse. Unless these fields are examined, a significant number of completed suicides could be missed, again flawing military medicine research.

8. Nonfatal suicide attempts. It is known that prior suicide attempts are the most valid predictors of future suicides, because an impulsive attempt that fails may not fail in future attempt(s). Paradoxically, most suicides seem not to have been intentional attempts to end one's life, but attempts at self-medication through powerful pharmaceuticals that, rather than dull the emotional pain, wind up killing the individual. These are called contraintentional and occur more with females overdosing on medications. In the military, quick access to lethal weapons is less likely to be contraintentional, although sometimes an intoxicated man will wake up with a gun pointed at his face. He may have passed out before "eating his gun" and pulling the trigger. This is less likely to happen with active duty soldiers, due to their 24/7 alertness and preparedness with a gun loaded and ready to fire at arm's length from them.

9. Suicidal Ideation—the vast majority of suicide cases discuss thoughts of suicide with doctors, caregivers, family, or friends within a few months of going through with it.

10. Depression and PTSD—researchers from Brigham Young University created a splash earlier this summer when they delivered a paper at a Defense Department conference, sharing research that affirms common wisdom: Soldiers try to kill themselves to end psychological pain. The study used data from interviews with seventy-two soldiers who are part of a larger three-year treatment

project at Fort Carson, Colorado. The seventy-two soldiers said they had tried to commit suicide or were suicidal because they wanted to stop bad feelings. While 10 percent said their suicide attempts were partially motivated by a desire to avoid an assignment or other issues, they also reported that they just wanted to end the suffering. Head project researcher, David Rudd, commented on the findings: "This provides . . . scientific backing that will help commanders and other service members understand that this is not someone trying to get out of something," he said, referring to the 90 percent of suicide attempts based on a soldier's unremitting state of hopelessness. The paper has been accepted for publication in the Journal of Affective Disorders. That means his findings associate emotional distress, or the mood disturbance of "dysphoria," as a necessary, if not sufficient, causative factor for suicide. This might also help explain the seemingly inexplicable crimes of Staff Sergeant Robert Bales, who, probably in pain and medicating himself with alcohol, sought a suicide by proxy, possibly to end his suffering.

Although the data compiled so far is seemingly self-evident, U.S. Army leadership is not all on the same page with such medical findings. A glaring example of that became public when Major General Dana Pittard, commanding general at Fort Bliss in Texas, wrote in his blog in January 2012. He told soldiers considering suicide to "act like an adult." General Pittard eventually retracted the statement, but did not apologize when, in a subsequent blog post, he said, "I have now come to the conclusion that suicide is an absolutely selfish act." He also wrote, "I am personally fed up with soldiers who are choosing to take their own lives so that others can clean up their messes. Be an adult, act like an adult, and deal with your real-life problems like the rest of us." He did also counsel soldiers to seek help.

Pittard's remarks drew a public rebuke from the Army, which has the highest number of suicides, and called his assertions "clearly wrong." The chairman of the Joint Chiefs of Staff, Army General

Martin Dempsey, said he disagrees with Pittard "in the strongest possible terms."

"The continual rise in the suicide rate has frustrated all in the military," says Elspeth "Cam" Ritchie, a retired Army colonel and chief psychiatric adviser to the Army Surgeon General. "The rise in the suicide rate continues despite numerous recommendations from the Army and [Department of Defense] task forces." She explained that suicide, and the reasons for it, have been a vexing problem for the U.S. military ever since its rate began eclipsing that of the U.S. population.

In 2010, the Army noted that, "historically, the suicide rate has been significantly lower in the military than among the U.S. civilian population." But that began to change as the wars in Afghanistan and Iraq, initially thought of by those who started them—but not by Colin Powell—as short-term affairs dragged on for years. More critical than their duration was the fact that, because we no longer had a universal draft (but rather a semi-privatized mercenary army), a relatively small number of U.S. troops kept being sent back for multiple combat tours. Repeated tours have driven up the rate of PTSD, which in turn generates an increase in suicide attempts among those suffering from PTSD. Although many troops who have killed themselves did not deploy, they trained amongst the dread of those who did. There is a sense, some service members say, that suicide, or at least suicide attempts, can be contagious. "There are two areas which we should explore further," says Ritchie, a regular Battleland contributor. "The high optempo [operations tempo] of deployed units, which means that leaders do not really know their soldiers; and the easy availability of firearms, the 'gun in the nightstand,' which, unfortunately, leads to too many impulsive suicides, and occasionally homicides.'"

10. Number of deployments with duration, both between and during deployment—Army research suggests that soldiers need at least two years of noncombat time before their symptoms of anxiety and

depression begin to wane. Reintegration can be a time of elevated risk for self-harm. Because the human survival mechanism, vital in combat, means that the body will secrete high amounts of adrenaline, there has to be a form of depressurization upon return from combat. Absent this controlled reintegration, soldiers who have high amounts of adrenaline coursing through their systems take high risks, which sometimes lead to accidents and other calamities.

Traditionally, the military has relied on suicide-mitigation strategies, such as buddy aid, where one soldier might notice unusual behavior in another and recommend he go for help.

"I'm not saying these have not worked," Dr. Ritchie said. "It's hard to know what would have happened otherwise, but it's clear [they're] not working well enough."

According to Utah researcher David Rudd at BYU, "It used to be that serving in the military made one less likely to commit suicide. Several years of war in the Middle East, when units were deploying two, three, four times, changed that."

Backing him up on that was testimony from leading military medicine experts and field commanders from the War on Terror. In morning testimony before the House Veterans Affairs Subcommittee on Health, Colonel Charles W. Hoge, M.D., Director of the Division of Psychiatry and Neuroscience at Walter Reed Army Institute of Research, said studies show "longer deployments, multiple deployments, greater time away from base camps, and combat intensity all contribute to higher rates of PTSD, depression, and marital problems." All of these are known risk factors for suicide in all populations.

Appearing later the very same afternoon before the Senate Armed Services Committee, Army Vice Chief of Staff General Richard Cody stated, "Today's Army is out of balance. The current demand for our forces in Iraq and Afghanistan exceeds the sustainable supply and limits our ability to provide ready forces for other contingencies. Current operational requirements for forces and insufficient time between deployments require a focus on counterinsurgency training and equipping to the detriment of preparedness for the full range of military missions. Given the current theater demand for Army forces, we are unable to provide a sustainable tempo of deployments for our soldiers and families."

Four-month rotations remain the standard for most Pacific airmen, but many are away for longer stretches. The wars in Iraq and Afghanistan were the first in which F-16CJ fighter jets were tasked to fly close-air support, providing cover, reconnaissance, and munitions to coalition ground forces. The military leaders' testimony at a Senate Armed Services subcommittee hearing fit a pattern of increasingly blunt warnings from the Pentagon about the war's toll on military families and equipment. Captaine Wes Ticer writes in Air Force Link: "Airmen from the 379th Air Expeditionary Wing continue to maintain increased operations, both in the air and on the ground, in support of ground forces in Afghanistan and Iraq. The 34th Expeditionary Bomb Squadron is called upon daily to provide close-air support to ground forces through precision bombing and shows of force and presence. The additional flying made for a busy week for aircrews and ground support." One can imagine how important precision is in the deployment of 500 bombs.

"This was a good test for us to stretch our legs a little and get a taste of Surge operations," said Lieutenant Colonel Quinten Miklos, the 34th EBS director of operations. "It's an issue of stamina because what I'm asking people to do is to fly sorties more frequently."

Aircrew members are on a cycle that consists of crew rest, flying, and recovering from a mission. A twelve-hour sortie typically occupies the aircrew for eighteen hours, Colonel Miklos said. "For the crews, it presents a scheduling challenge, because we are limited in the normal flow of sortie generation. Our planners have to juggle the schedule to adjust crews to ensure the proper rest and time for planning."

At sea, things are stretched thin, too. "There are almost 1,400 Pacific Fleet sailors serving as individual augmentees in CENTCOM, with hundreds more at sea, the Navy said. The deployments range from six months to a year. Navy leaders want to strike a better balance between War on Terror requirements and improving stability for sailors and families at home," said Petty Officer First Class Shane Tuck, a Pacific Fleet spokesman. "A new detailing process will be used for permanent-change-of-station transfers, rather than a 'midtour, short-notice assignment,'" he added. But was this done?

11. Male Sexual Trauma (MST)—most victims of MST make suicidal attempts, and most MST is immensely underreported. Soldiers are to remain totally celibate during fifteen months of deployment, unless fortunate enough to have consensual intimacy with another soldier, whether gay, lesbian, or heterosexual. Females deploying are less than 10 percent of the force. There are no figures on LBGT. But to fraternize intimately with locals is against military regulation. Is it surprising that sexual assault is showing its ugly head after nearly a dozen years of war with nearly three million men and women at the prime of their active sexual lives deployed as, what Ambassador Crocker described, "strangers" on foreign soil? Ambassador Crocker is deeply skeptical that "Americans on foreign soil can be anything other than strangers in a strange land."

"Male veterans who have a history of military sexual trauma often fail to disclose their condition until well into treatment for Post-Traumatic Stress Disorder and have many motivations for covering up their problem, according to speakers at the annual meeting of the International Society for Traumatic Stress Studies. Another complication is that few clinicians know of community resources to whom to refer male military sexual trauma (MST) patients," said Ilona L. Pivar, Ph.D., of the National Center for Post-Traumatic Stress Disorder in the Veterans Affairs Palo Alto healthcare System.

"When you're sexually traumatized in the military by other veterans, combat veterans sometimes don't believe you and may in fact mock you," Dr. Kathleen Chard said. Dr. Chard is the director of the PTSD and Anxiety Disorders Division at the Cincinnati VA Medical Center and an associate professor of clinical psychiatry at the University of Cincinnatti. Some VA residential trauma programs across the country also have been accused of saying things like: "We'll only take you through combat trauma, and if you have other types of trauma, we may allow you to talk about that privately if there's time and therapist availability."

"When I heard that, I immediately made a decision that we're going to change our modality," Dr. Chard said.

Now any veteran with PTSD from any event, such as child abuse, MST, or combat trauma, is welcome in the VA residential treatment programs. Dr. Chard says, "I'm not saying that we're the best model, but we're the model that fits the needs of Cincinnati veterans at the time, and with this response: Referrals have gone up about 25 percent since we created this change." Dr. I. Pivar, a specialist in dealing with anxiety, grief, and PTSD in returning combat veterans added, "I speak from experience, because of the difficulty getting referrals [and] the difficulty educating providers, that this is a problem, and that I am there as a resource for referrals," In a sample of thirty male veterans with MST who were treated at the Cincinnati VA residential treatment program over an 18-month period, only three divulged their MST at the outset. Their MST had not been identified in any pretreatment notes at their home VA before coming to the Cincinnati VA. All met criteria for MST at some point in treatment. The veterans served in the Vietnam War (18), the post-Vietnam War era (9), and in the first Gulf War (3). Contributing factors to the low awareness of MST among men include shame and stigma and resistance to being labeled or targeted as a victim of MST. These are perpetuated by myths about male sexual assault, such as the notion that males cannot be raped, sexual assaults against men happen only in prison, male adult victims must be homosexual, heterosexual males do not rape men, and males are less affected by sexual assault than are females.

"I have veterans who I've treated who do not want to have that box in the VA system checked 'MST,' and they don't have it [checked]; however, they have MST and they have PTSD," Dr. Kathleen Chard said. "Their initial treatment in the military may have been a precursor for this kind of sensitivity. Certainly, my veterans who are older experienced this as 'something that doesn't happen,' and are told to keep it quiet or are moved away to another unit or even punished."

The types of sexual trauma, focused on males as well as females, include unexpected sexual overtures that are disruptive to self-identity, assault during or after combat (such as an assault by a medic), assault while in military prison, and being targeted by a person higher in command or being assaulted for being weak or small. Possible clues to identifying MST in men include substance abuse (which is often severe), problems with sexual intimacy, difficulties with male relationships, marital relationship problems, problems with authority, fear of being labeled homosexual or sexually impotent, history of child sexual abuse or exposure to abuse, anger and aggression, and a history of violence.

The VA does have an effective screening program, but some patients are missed because of stigma and shame. Unless delicately and routinely explored, a veteran can keep this trauma a secret for decades. If veterans finally reveal MST, they are often surprised to learn that other male soldiers have experienced sexual trauma as well. Dr. Pivar presented a small pilot study of ten male veterans from all military service branches who had experienced MST at a mean age of twenty years. Men were the perpetrators, except for one veteran who had been assaulted by two women. Nine males were heterosexual, while one was bisexual. Six have tried to commit suicide or self-harm as teenagers or adults, and all had severe substance abuse problems following their MST. ("VA Data Reinforce Need for Treatment of Sexual Trauma," CLINICAL PSYCHIATRY NEWS, January 2008 and Clinical Psychiatry News, 03/01/08)

13. Quality of Weaponry—It should not be an issue, but shockingly and disgustingly, it is. As reported in Senate testimony, "Soldiers, families, support systems, and equipment are stretched and stressed by the demands of lengthy and repeated deployments, with insufficient recovery time. Equipment used repeatedly in harsh environments is wearing out more rapidly than programmed. Amy support systems, designed for the pre-September 11th peacetime Army, are straining under the accumulation of stress from six years at war. Overall, our readiness is being consumed as fast as we build it. If unaddressed, this lack of balance poses a significant risk to the All-Volunteer Force and degrades the Army's ability to make a timely response to other contingencies." Senate Armed Services Committee testimony, Army Vice Chief of Staff G. Richard Cody.

In discussing transformation of military logistics in Operation Enduring Freedom for the press, it was stated, "In the past, most of the Army prepositioned stocks were intended for high-end combat operation. Army officials acknowledge that, in decades past, they have allowed weapons prepositioned for combat to become badly outdated." In a *New York Times* report, it was revealed that when the first troops reached Kuwait for the 2003 Iraq invasion, the tanks and armored vehicles were inferior to the equipment the soldiers had trained on. They were required to "train down" for the invasion in order to reduce waiting to attack and spending money to replace old inventory with newer and safer vehicles shipped from the U.S. (*New York Times*, 7/27/12). And according to Navy psychiatrists at Twentynine Palms, Marines are deploying so frequently that their weapons cannot be maintained.

In the case of Charles at Khe Sanh, Vietnam: "I was on clean-up duty and came across the remains of a firefight. It was a Marine patrol, and they were slaughtered. The NVA stripped them of everything but their weapons and ammo. I noticed the ammo was "blue dot" from the Korean War inventory. The enemy knew this, because their weapons had jammed."

Are such fraudulent procurement, contracting, and logistics impacting force protection, as is apparently the case with recurrent six-month deployments of Twentynine Palms Marine units? Possibly. Why would The War on Terror make military procurement, contracting, and logistics more honest than in any other war?

14. Separations and losses, both in combat and at home, have spurred suicides and family violence. In some cases, soldiers, like the Thomas Stroh case cited previously, have committed murders of their spouses and even their children before killing themselves. Some experts believe this is the direct result of multiple deployments, which place families and spouses under great strain that they are unable to cope with. It can be incredibly difficult to tolerate a spouse, boyfriend, or girlfriend who cannot express emotions and be emotionally supportive over a long period of time. Eventually, partners of those suffering from PTSD lose hope in their loved one's ability to return to their old selves. So they get out of the relationship. Separations and rejections in such intimate relations are frequently triggering events for veterans, whether active duty soldiers or one-time Special Operations stars like suicidal murderer Dr. Timothy Jorden in Buffalo, or Sikh Temple suicidal mass murderer Wade Page in Milwaukee. Both of the latter two catastrophic murder-suicides were closely associated with rejection and separation from girlfriends.

15. Survival Guilt, Transgressions, and Shame—Many soldiers who feel guilty about surviving or feel shame for having transgressed in some way take it out on themselves and often their families. In the cases of Sergeant David Stewart and Thomas Stroh—both of

whom died in car crashes, and both of whose families were later discovered to have been murdered in their homes—there was an eerie similarity. Stewart, who underwent several medical procedures, seemed to descend into a deep depression, just like Stroh. In cases involving deep depression—a depression in which the sufferer feels hopeless, sees no value in living, and believes that death is the only way to relieve his emotional pain—the sufferer may often take his family with him in a final act of annihilation. The questions raised in the case of Army medic David Stewart opens the shades on the often chaotic battlefield of Operation Enduring Freedom. Why was he feeling guilt? What were his transgressions? Before taking his life, he wrote to friends of impending prosecution. For what? Was he in real criminal trouble, or psychotically depressed with delusions and hallucinations of extreme guilt over doing something for which he was not really responsible? He also referred to "secrets;" what "secrets" should buddies be on the alert to?

Contrast the experiences of combat veterans from the wars in Iraq and Afghanistan with the experiences of the G.I.s in World War II, who fought well-armed, well-led, and ferocious Japanese and German armies. As they penetrated deeper into enemy territory, they began to see more and more of the atrocities committed by the totalitarian regimes of the Axis leaders. The slaves working in "work camps," and then the horrors of genocide in death camps and Asian POW camps, infuriated them and motivated them to fight forward. Most considered their chances of returning home to be slim. There was usually one deployment, and it continued until VE and VJ days. There was, however, a front line and secure rear areas, mostly populated with grateful, liberated civilians. They could look forward to rest and relaxation in these friendly communities, which were secured and already starting to rebuild for the future. War brides were discovered. Their cause was unequivocally just. Their mission clear. The fight was worth it, although none would say any war's cause is worth very much more than sacrifice of life, limb, and human ideals. Nothing is like that in Operation Enduring Freedom; nor was anything like that in *Operation Iraqi Freedom*. The purposes of these wars are not clear, and often it was difficult to discern who were the good guys, and who were the bad. If our political and military leaders know the answers to the why of these missions, they have kept them from both the public and most certainly from the troops. Bin Laden is dead. Iraq, on close inspection, had no weapons of mass destruction.

Robert Jay Lifton, in his pioneering work on the returning Vietnam veteran (*Home from the War: Learning from Vietnam Veterans*, Other Press, 2005), asked the basic question all clinicians raised in those deaf and dumb clinical days of the Vietnam War, when combat histories were rarely taken on VA patients, and the diagnosis of Post-Traumatic Stress Disorder did not even exist. Dr. Lifton, however, was a scholar in the field of extreme trauma and addressed the issue by interviewing returning Vietnam veterans. It must be remembered that the Army medical policy for draftees deployed to Vietnam was essentially, "Anyone can take anything for a year." It was a self-delusion; a fallacy that affected an entire generation of American veterans.

Army psychiatrist Colonel Franklyn Jones traveled the world at the government's expense, touting the accomplishments of cutting psychiatric evacuation rates from Vietnam from 22 percent in the Korean War to 1 percent in the Vietnam War. He probably took the illusion to his grave that his policy of "immediacy and expectancy" increased the resilience of these young draftees. Symptoms of crying, screaming, or going mute, all evidence of some form of emotional trauma and residual mental illness, would not get you out of Vietnam. Who made up the 1 percent evacuated to Japan? Probably overtly psychotic soldiers who were an imminent threat to others or an extreme drain on resources. Colonel Jones's policies, despite miraculous statistical achievement in military medicine, were total failures—although enduring achievements for him, at least among his superiors who didn't need to address traumatic neurosis in Vietnam veterans.

Lifton obviously ignored Colonel Jones's politicized whitewash of the day and dug into the combat experiences of those who Jones might have called "whiners" and "malingerers." Almost universally in returning vets, he found survivor guilt and a profound sense of transgression incompatible with these young draftees' moral identities; young men were mostly raised in church back then. Lifton's new preface connects the experience of Vietnam veterans with that of veterans of the war in Iraq. Both were brought into the "atrocity-producing situations" that led to My Lai and Abu Ghraib. Lifton raises the possibility that Iraq veterans could experience the kind of healing transformation that many who fought in Vietnam were able to achieve.

In an article in Nervous Mental Disease, H.J. Glover says that the guilt that combat veterans suffer from in its most acute form resembles "agitated depression." Events that took place during combat can create feelings of survival guilt, the feelings of which stem from the group camaraderie of a tight-knit military unit, especially at a forward operating base in which soldiers are protective of each other. That protectiveness bestows a sense of control over the situation. Consequently, when one of the soldiers dies in violent combat, the other soldiers can feel failure, guilt, or sink into a deep depression, which can be suicidal. Soldiers who had difficult childhoods may reexperience old feelings of guilt and become even more susceptible to deep intractable depression and consequent suicidal ideations. (Nerv Ment Dis 172: 393-397, 1988).

This description very accurately describes the feelings of more than one soldier who has felt guilt, remorse, and shame over the troops he lost at forward operating bases or other outposts in Afghanistan—troops they had to protect, and troops who protected them. Soldiers may still feel this guilt at having failed to protect their buddies in combat even after they have returned home and read reports of soldiers who have died in battle.

In a study of military suicides, entitled Soul Repair: Recovering from Moral Injury After War (Beacon, November 2012), co-authors Colonel Herman Keizer, Jr. (co-director of the Soul Repair Center, who served for thiry-four years as a military chaplain), and Dr. Gabriella Lettini suggest that the most serious blind spot in the reporting on military suicides is an absence of discussions about the moral impact of military training and its implementation in combat. Soldiers, they write, are trained to kill, which is regarded as criminal behavior in civilian life, and they are trained to be lethal without even thinking about it; a method of training called "reflexive fire." They suggest that moral injury, not PTSD, is likely one of the most important factors in military suicides, because moral guilt slowly sinks into a veteran's psyche. Unlike soldiers with preexisting psychiatric conditions—or even those having emerged from abusive childhoods—moral injury has its greatest effect on an otherwise healthy brain because that soldier can feel empathy towards those he has killed. Because that soldier can evaluate his own behavior, he experiences what the authors call a "negative self-judgment," resulting from a transgression of his "core moral beliefs." There is a consequent decay and deterioration of the soldier's "moral identity." He feels betrayed by superiors who ordered him to kill. This, in turn, results in his feeling shame and survivor guilt, dropping into substance addiction, and ultimately slipping into a depression that can be lethal to himself and others.

The Army, although it trains soldiers to survive and to fight, also places its soldiers in these ill-conceived forays into insurgent civilian populations. The soldier's survival mechanism, and his protective embrace of members of his unit, means that the solder will turn his fire on civilians who, he believes, pose a threat to his life and mission. But turning fire on civilians is a violation of the soldier's moral standards, as well as international law. In World War II, the victorious Allies executed German and Japanese commanders who committed atrocities. However, in the Middle East, and before that in Vietnam, we counted civilian victims in body counts because we couldn't tell for sure who were the enemy insurgents and who were the innocent civilians. Soldiers with even a moderate moral upbringing would, of course, suffer guilt if they believed they were killing innocent civilians. Keizer and Lentinni write that the very act of placing soldiers among a civilian population in a counter-insurgency war puts those soldiers at the risk of debilitating and often fatal mental illness as the result of shame, guilt, and the need for self-punishment (Soul Repair: Recovering from Moral Injury After War, (Beacon November 2012).

The most recent Army attempt to prepare troops for battle appears to have failed miserably. Its "Comprehensive Soldier Fitness" (CSF) program, begun in 2009 with a $125 million investment and lauded in a *New York Times* article in March 2012, has been widely criticized. It bypasses the difficult ethical questions that many healthy human beings ask about war, and its spiritual fitness component has no moral content. It suggests that a soldier's commitment to a higher purpose—mission first—makes for resiliency. But most people capable of such a commitment also have empathy for others and deep moral values.

The Army's "spiritual fitness" encourages soldiers to see events in a neutral light, rather than labeling them as good or bad, and to create a nightly list of positive things that happened that day. The lack of awareness is startling regarding what it might mean to ask someone to think of killing a child, losing a close friend, or torturing detainees as a neutral or positive event. Proving a direct cause-effect relationship between such training and suicides is difficult, of course. However, there are certain moral reactions to war and the experience of combat training that indicate a violation of moral conscience, which can have devastating consequences for soldiers' psyches.

The reporting on military and veteran suicides mostly fails to explore the role of moral injury. When a suicide occurs years after a soldier returns from war, combat experience is often disregarded as a primary cause of the suicide. Yet, as Karl Marlantes, a Vietnam veteran, reports in *What It Is Like to Go to War,* he was fine for a decade, and then he crashed. Often, such delays are used to deny VA services or are regarded as a family problem, rather than as a consequence of service in combat. We can see how this skews the medical morbidity statistics on suicide causation and its relationship to the combat experience.

The alarming rates of reported suicides are squishy statistics and do not reflect the true numbers of soldiers who take their own lives. Many combat veterans tell stories of comrades who shot themselves, but who were reported as "non-combat" or "accidental" casualties. Soldiers who deliberately place themselves in harm's way in hopes of dying are reported as casualties, not suicides, which is what might have happened to Sergeant Bales had he been successful in his attempt at suicide-by-proxy in Afghanistan. Since many life insurance policies will not pay benefits to families if suicide is the cause of death, the need to disguise suicide may mean some apparently accidental deaths were, in actuality, planned. We will never know the true suicide numbers, but we do speculate from the cases we have seen that many seemingly accidental fatalities were indeed suicides.

16. Pre-military psychiatric and medical history—Completion of basic training and deployment does not screen out young men with genetic risks of suicide or even Bipolar Affective Disorder (Manic Depressive Disease), which is highly genetically determined and common. But risk factors for suicide among a military population can differ from the general population. The typical soldier at risk of suicide does not have a long history of mental health issues. What we don't see is major mental illness, such as Schizophrenia or Bipolar Disorder, that is disabling. Only about 5 percent of military suicides are associated with a diagnosis of personality disorders,

which is "lower than I would have expected," said former Army chief psychiatrist Dr. Elspeth Ritchie, a retired colonel, who also is a professor of psychiatry at Uniformed Services University of the Health Sciences, in Bethesda, Maryland.

17. Comorbid TBI with loss of impulse control and ability to cope with challenges of daily living—Colonel Elspeth Ritchie has argued that, "Effective interventions in a military population will require a comprehensive look at all the elements around suicide, including Post-Traumatic Stress Disorder (PTSD), mild Traumatic Brain Injury (TBI), and depression." According to Colonel Ritchie, the type of warfare many soldiers see when deployed in Afghanistan or Iraq increases their risk for mild TBI and associated symptoms. "The signature weapon of this war is the blast. And that causes a lot of symptoms." Reexperiencing the trauma, numbing/avoidance, and physiologic arousal ("flight-or-fight" response) are the three main PTSD symptom clusters.

18. Chronic Pain Syndrome, commonly associated with both depression and combat PTSD—Chronic pain, especially if left untreated for a year or more, can lead to depression and the sufferer's ultimate self-destructive conclusion that suicide is the only way out of pain. Therefore, chronic pain must be appreciated as a contributory factor in self-inflicted fatalities.

19. Access to Care and Willingness to Seek Help—The mere act of seeking mental help for self can be perceived as a sign of weakness. Unfortunately, and despite the horrifying statistics of one Army suicide each day, many senior officers at the top of the command chain still do not grasp the seriousness of this problem. This is why the Army Surgeon General Horoho promised Senator Patty Murray that the Army would investigate and remediate in the closure of the Madigan intensive psychotherapy clinic for PTSD. Recent headlines

in the *Seattle Times* speak of betrayal, possibly from the very top of Army command. So what should the average soldier, already distressed and at his or her wit's end, read into this command action at one of the largest and most central military medical facilities for our War on Terror?

Perhaps it is best to stay away from so-called behavioral health clinics like these. Their credibility of being in the soldier's best interest is just one more flashing sign to the survivor of betrayal awaiting again—this time titled "behavioral health."

Study co-director of STARRS, Dr. Robert J. Ursano (professor of psychiatry and neuroscience, chair of the Department of Psychiatry, and director of the Center for the Study of Traumatic Stress at the Uniformed Services University of the Health Sciences in Bethesda), supports the empirical goals of suicide research in the military, and said that the researchers will eventually draw on massive datasets covering thousands of soldiers—again, presumably only enlisted men, to the exclusion of National Guardsmen and activated reservists. "This is an early cross-sectional look at single variables that leaves us with a number of potential explanations. There are limitations attached to the data released now, but there is always a challenge between science and the need for making decisions about national security," Ursano has said. Translated, this means that we cannot have force protection without force health protection. Suicidal soldiers and officers are a threat to the missions on foreign soil, specifically because suicidal individuals can also commit ancillary violence, as in the case of Robert Bales.

Suicide is a key focus of the National Center for Veterans Studies, where psychologist researchers oversee projects that are teasing out causes and determining the best treatments for combat PTSD. The research is funded by the Department of Defense, which in recent years has poured millions of dollars into the confounding issue of active-duty suicides. Between 1998 and 2011, a June report showed that 2,990 servicemen and women died by suicide. The number per year nearly doubled between 2005 and 2009, when it peaked at about 290. The statistics were published in the *Medical Surveillance Monthly Report*, a publication of the Armed Forces Health Surveillance Center. When the number of active-duty armed service members taking their own lives dropped slightly in 2010—and again in 2011—the Pentagon took it as a sign that its prevention efforts were paying off. This year, however, suicides are on the rise again.

The Pentagon announced in June that 154 active-duty soldiers, sailors, airmen, and Marines took their own lives in the first 155 days of the year, outnumbering those killed in combat in Afghanistan. The National Center for Veterans Studies is convinced that the way the nation wages war and the nature of these wars—guerilla warfare, where warriors often can't tell the difference between combatants and civilians—is to blame. The Center's research indicates that because the nature of war has changed, psychological injury is the "most significant consequence" because of its disproportionate impact upon surviving veterans. And because psychological injuries are not palpable or visible surface injuries, such as bullet wounds, even sufferers initially see their mental illness as a form of weakness. Real men don't complain or run for help from psychiatrists. And as a result, the illness metastasizes and can become lethal.

More specific to the assigned unit and its combat history as a risk factor, new research at the University of Utah's National Center for Veterans Studies shows that the more severe combat a warrior experiences, the more likely he or she is to later attempt suicide. For those in the center's study of 244 soldiers who saw heavy combat, the findings are stark: 93 percent qualified for a diagnosis of Post-Traumatic Stress Disorder, and nearly 70 percent had attempted suicide. Colonel Carl Castro, who oversees the Department of Defense's research into suicide prevention and treatment, says the center's findings contribute to a growing body of research into the "tremendous psychological and physical burden" that combat places on service members.

Suicide research has, and still continues to be, poorly funded when compared to other medical conditions. This is particularly problematic, given that suicide is one of the top-ten causes of death in the United States and the second leading cause for young people. The Deparment of Defense and VA-funded research underway in the past decade, however, will (clinicians hope) advance the entire mental health profession with respect to the understanding of traumatic stress and PTSD, particularly PTSD suffered as a result of combat.

Because the severity of psychiatric symptoms relates directly to the severity of the combat experience, it puts to rest the notion that warriors become more resilient and more comfortable the longer they are in combat. That's a bromide sometimes used by those who dismiss combat as a cause because, after all, roughly half of the suicides occur among military members who never leave the United States. David Rudd of the Veteran's Center study at Brigham Young argues that noncombat veteran suicides are a separate issue. What his research indicates, he says, is that there are two separate groups of veterans, with two separate sets of suicidal causalities.

Compounding the findings of Rudd are the research findings and theory of suicide causation of clinical psychologists Craig J. Bryan, PsyD, and Kelly C. Cukrowicz, PhD, published in *Suicide and Life-Threatening Behavior* 41(2) in April 2011 and presented before The American Association of Suicidology. They found that combat exposure might increase risk in proportion to the severity of the traumatic exposures to painful and provocative experiences as a result of defensive survival responses, such as fearlessness about death and increased pain tolerance. They theorized that the severity of exposure and extremity of such survival defenses enhances the individual's capability to attempt suicide. Thus, surviving the most violent and aggressive combat experiences demonstrate relatively stronger associations to capacity for completing suicide. It sounds paradoxical on the surface, but it's true and potentially frightening, not only for the military, but for society in general.

They tested their proposition in a sample of deployed active duty combatants and found that all types of combat exposure independently contribute to a capability for suicide. Conceptualizing their study within the construct of interpersonal-psychological theory of suicide (IPTS), when considering all types of combat simultaneously, combat characterized by violence and high levels of injury and death are associated with relatively stronger associations to capability for completing suicide. Surprisingly few studies have tried to connect the type and intensity of the trauma—or what might be considered the "dose"—to risk of completing suicide. Bryan and Cukrowicz found that combat experiences with marked exposure to pain, injury, death, and aggression contribute to suicidal behaviors "through the dual processes of habituation to the fear of death and increased tolerance for pain. These two processes comprise the capability for suicide." This was inside the military, but if you stretch this by analogy to police in violent and lethal shootouts, disaster workers, and even at-risk children exposed to exceptionally bloody simulations in violent video games, you can see the direction this takes us.

These findings are similar to studies of suicidality from childhood abuse, where more intense levels of physical pain such as rape and physical abuse are better predictors of subsequent suicidal behavior than less physically painful forms of childhood abuse, such as molestation and verbal abuse (Joiner et al., 2007). "Based on the IPTS's assumptions that fearlessness about death is a necessary condition for suicidal intent to emerge, and higher levels of pain tolerance are required for more highly lethal suicidal behaviors, Van Orden et al. (2010) have proposed that the capability for suicide contributes directly to suicidal intent and lethality of suicidal behaviors. This is consistent with empirical findings demonstrating that an increased sense of courage or perceived competence about suicide is more closely related to suicidal behaviors than the desire for death or suicide (Beck, Brown, & Steer, 1997; Joiner, Rudd, &

Rajab, 1997), generally due to their close association with other factors, such as access to lethal means, mental rehearsal, preparation for death, and behavioral practice of the suicide method, all of which habituate the individual to the fearsome act of lethal or near-lethal suicidal behavior."

When viewed through the lens of the IPTS, the finding that violent or aggressive combat events are more strongly associated with later suicide attempts than less violent combat events (Fontana et al., 1992) has provided a possible explanatory mechanism: habituation to death and increased pain tolerance. Results of the current study are consistent with the possibility that Fontana et al.'s findings are due to an increased exposure to more violent combat experiences. What might be a fascinating corollary study would be to look at earlier warlike cultures, particularly in medieval through nineteenth-century Japan, where suicide was a ritual; or in Anglo-Saxon heroic poetry culture, where suicide by proxy was considered a virtue, as long as the warrior took his enemies with him.

In light of Bryan's results, is he studying a different group of combat veterans whose pain is so excruciating that suicide is the only means of relief, because Bryan and Cukrowicz's study subjects are more numb? Not necessarily, because the human brain's response to extreme psychological trauma is to activate its own opiates. Van der Kolk demonstrated this in comparing Vietnam veterans, who were in intense combat, with non-combatant Vietnam veterans, and adjusted for all other factors possible, including race, religion, age, and cultural background. He tested this out in an almost *Stanley Kubrickian's Clockwork Orange way*. While showing vivid combat scenes from the Oliver Stone motion picture *Platoon* to his test subjects, Van der Kolk found that combat veterans numbed themselves to the pain of pricking their skin with a needle, but non-combatants did not. Even more significant was the finding that this numbing response from the brain's own opiate secretion in response to trauma was eliminated with the administration of an opiate-blocking drug, Naltrexone. These study results pose the question: Are the subjects who numbed themselves more likely to complete a suicidal act than those who are in so much emotional pain that suicide is the only way out?

The probable answer is that these are the same subjects. Veterans exposed to high doses of violence, death, and horrors of war survived by numbing themselves and also generating other brain chemicals such as cortisone. Van der Kolk's patients are not necessarily numb all the time, thus facing and habituated to more exposure to traumatic cues. They numb, but numbing does not necessarily mean they are not in emotional distress. His subjects simply did not feel the physical pain of being stuck with a needle. Similarly, survivors of severe child abuse will cut themselves to generate their opiates. We have found from therapy interviews that they may do this to reduce their emotional pain, called "dysphoria" (as compared to "euphoria," which is feeling high). This is a compulsion to repeat their traumatic experience, or what might be called "habituation" in the context of IPTS theory of Bryan and Cukrowicz's subjects, who are not necessarily high as if on Demerol. If you've taken Demerol after deep gum periodontal surgery, for example, you may recall that you feel the pain, but you don't perceive it as intolerably distressing. So the self-cutter who experienced such severe pain when raped at a young age has the compulsion to repeat the trauma and reexperience her numbing to it as defense to repeated rape. This is not to be confused with feeling either well or euphoric on dope. Self-cutters do not feel good before they cut, and they don't feel well when they cut. But when they cut, they can reexperience the childhood rape with the numbing. So in the same way, is the patient who is so dysphonic he cannot take it anymore, but can nonetheless re-experience the horrific faces of combat with the numbing and courage to face death, including his own. Death may not always take the seriously suicidal soldier. Rather, Bryan and Cukrowicz's subjects courageously overcome the ultimate threat of their own destruction, but on their own terms and with their own bullets. In this study, they demonstrate that they have found a way around their own destruction, albeit via a form of dysfunctional or self destructive behaviors that reexperience the pain, as in cutting or hanging oneself.

In the 1970s, the Vietnam veterans returned home from the war to hostile peers who did not go. They might have been exempted from the draft, like a Mitt Romney or a Bill Clinton, because the draft created a two-tier class of young men: Those who could get out, and those who had to take their places. But many of those who could get out called the vets "baby killers." They were so called by high school classmates who did not go and became protestors against the war. There were also academics, those who'd gotten student deferments through college and graduate school, who opposed the war, berated the veterans, and protested them when they came home, which was why any formal acknowledgment of Vietnam War vets' service had to wait for an entire decade.

The only thing most of the protestors and veterans had in common was drugs. Heroin and hash were high quality in Vietnam. Pot, too, was primo and in abundance. Getting stoned or tripping out on LSD, as Francis Ford Coppola so brilliantly depicted in *Apocalypse Now*, was a daily routine for many of the screaming protestors at home, especially in college dorms during the late 1960s, as well as for many veterans both in theater and at home. Remember, not only was LSD part of a military intelligence experiment in the 1950s— with former Army Intelligence (G-2) commanding general Arthur Trudeau slipping it into the morning coffee of the U.S. Army General Staff—but even the CIA was supplying it to President Kennedy at the White House via Timothy Leary to both Mary Pinchot Meyer and Dr. Max Jacobson. That was then.

This is now: The nearly three million veterans of multiple tours in the War on Terror are not coming home to their peers demonstrating on the streets and calling them baby killers when they walk out of their bases to reintegrate to home life. They are coming home to silence, as if the war never happened. Glad you folks are home, get a job. Only there are no jobs. There is only silence, and the echoes of trauma from combat that nobody else seems to appreciate or recognize. This is like the disavowal of incest; the second injury of denial. Nobody on the news in the apocalyptic death of officers and Christopher Dorner ever brought up the question, "What did Dorner experience in Iraq?" Is it of any interest? It wasn't to the LAPD. And if it wasn't of any interest, is that not a disavowal of the trauma experienced by this generation of volunteers sent repeatedly to combat Muslim extremists who attacked us on September 11th?

How do they interpret their mission, now that it is essentially over, but without any sign of mission accomplished? Just debate over whether it should have occurred in the first place? The silence over this mission and its combat wounded is deafening from peers and family who did not volunteer. Do we really want to know why Christopher Dorner was crying in his patrol car and pleading for reintegration training following another deployment to Iraq? Do we really want to know what led up to the creation of a monster named Seargant Robert Bales? It appears not; especially at Madigan, where claims of disability resulting from battlefield trauma and associated disorders were denied by psychiatrists functioning as insurance claims adjusters.

In advocating for Department of Defense-mandated annual and post-deployment screening for suicide that enhances access to care, Dr. Elspeth Ritchie said, "There is a reassessment three to six months after they come back, because they may not be truthful right after deployment." She adds, by way of explanation, that the Army leadership acknowledges that some personnel might minimize their feelings immediately post-combat to expedite their return home. This means that even if they do have access to mental health counseling, they won't seek it. That's why Dr. Ritchie advocates mandated mental health assessment and screening. Combat veterans have discovered that a clean bill of health with no administrative loose ends will get them out of combat faster than if there were medical iterations they had to resolve. Accordingly, any veteran feeling pain and suffering would want to get out of the combat zone and back to safety, even if it meant cloaking feelings to get home and putting oneself at risk of greater mental decomposition and possible risk of suicide. Considering that possibility, the Department of Defense continues to develop and promote new suicide prevention initiatives. A task force aimed at reducing suicide is currently working on state-of-the-art, universal, multidisciplinary suicide awareness and prevention training. Technology aimed at augmenting therapy is another strategy, one designed to overcome some access to care issues in remote areas. Virtual reality programs and telemedicine are examples.

"Telemedicine is not a silver bullet," Dr. Ritchie said. "It is very time-intensive, but can be effective." Are these initiatives working? "It's a little early to tell. 2009 was an extraordinary year for suicide—the highest they have been," Dr. Ritchie said. And so was 2010. "It seems that it is lower so far this year [2012]. There is hope, Dr. Ritchie continued, that suicides will now be trending down. "We are holding our breath on that one."

In addition, she adds that the National Institute of Mental Health is funding a $50 million study, known as the Army Study, to assess risk and resilience in service members and the epidemiology of suicide. The challenge, according to Dr. Ritchie, is going to be using that epidemiology research to create effective suicide prevention programs. So how can this translational research be "actionable," as is the term our military requires to inform both strategy and tactics?

By integrating the analytics of clinical decision-making into AHLTA, clinicians could be limited in what diagnoses they enter, especially if they are not yet certain of the specifics of their diagnoses. Entering "Depression NOS," for example, informs clinicians of almost nothing, as was the case when Cho Seung-Hui was discharged back to the Virginia Tech campus after a brief involuntary detention in the local hospital with the diagnosis of Depression NOS. That diagnosis turned out to be fatal, because it might have described every other student on the VT campus after a bad date, a drunken night on the town, and a severe headache on Sunday morning. In other words, a diagnosis of Depression NOS is, more often than not, almost useless.

When prescribing a medication on AHLTA, the prescriber cannot submit any drug to the pharmacist until he reviews potential interactions with drugs that the patient currently takes, potential adverse reactions of the drug, and then decides to push the "override" button. This makes the clinician at least think about prescribing a drug that could increase the metabolic destruction of another critical drug, possibly impairing the treatment efforts of another physician. Such discipline should be built into AHLTA for reducing the risk of missing potentially lethal mental states of unremitting human destructiveness. Since many of these cross- and contra-indicators for medications are already built into many large pharmaceutical software programs, it should be a fix we can make through Computer Aided Diagnostics (CAD).

Certainly, no clinician can predict violent acts to self, others, or both with 100 percent certainty, and they must respect the patient's rights. There must be—as Miller proves with research on CAD— discipline in the clinicians' search for risk factors of suicides when the uncommon opportunity of interviewing a soldier presents itself. It has been proven that every physician needs more information every day of his practice than is stored in the best of clinicians' brains. Yet robotics and computers are not all that is needed. They are tools. There is no substitute for face-to-face clinical interviews by competent and experienced clinicians, if the current epidemic of suicides is to be nipped in the bud. It can be done, but it will require clinically intelligent medical software development for AHLTA as fail-safe, as is the e-prescribing described, requiring the clinician to confirm reading the risks of prescriptive powers before overriding based on clinical judgment, personal knowledge, and experience. In other words, the clinical encounter with a patient potentially at risk for suicide or violence because of mental illness must begin by eliminating various risk factors. That means, first of all, immediately ruling out the risk of causing harm to the medical evaluator himself, followed by the immediate risk of the patient harming himself and imminent risks for harming others. As we outline in our best practices algorithm below, aligning the rules of the DSM with triage protocols and interviewing patients presenting with depression, as labor-intensive as that may be, stands the greatest chance of preventing suicide among our combat personnel and veterans.

Chapter 10

Fixing Military and VA Health Care

President Dwight Eisenhower said in 1966, according to the *New York Times*: "Under the system that I envision, every young male American, no matter what status in life or plan for the future, would spend forty-nine weeks—one year, minus three weeks vacation—in military training. Only the barest minimum of exemptions would be permitted. Obviously mental impairment, those with some drastic defect, perhaps a few extreme hardship cases, qualify for deferment."

This statement best defines what our most important military leader and president believed about the military and national service. In some ways, Eisenhower, a diplomat and statesman as well as the commander-in-chief during World War II (who managed to amalgamate and keep together the Allied coalition by smoothing over differences and coordinating combined strategy), was a visionary about this country's needs. He also vehemently expressed skepticism of new wars, saying that every dollar spent on a round of ammunition was a dollar not spent on education. He won a war, kept us out of other wars and warned about the very military-industrial complex that we now have. This complex of industry and the Pentagon, along with foreign government lobbies, has not only worked us into a state of never-ending war that has dominated the first decade of the twenty-first century, but it has profited from these wars in ways that rise to corruption and are downright immoral.

Ike's vision for a citizen army—an army composed of draftees serving with no exceptions, except for the physically and mentally infirm—is not a vision that this nation embraced. In fact, the president who took us out of the draft was Ike's own vice president, Richard Nixon. After all, the thinking as the Vietnam War wore on was that if we had an all-volunteer army, there would be no pesky protests about wars college kids would be forced to fight. Nixon was right, but look where it got us.

We currently have a private mercenary army that can barely fight one war, much less two; an army that relies on National Guard, reserve troops, and private contractors, and which is subject to multiple deployments. We are looking at soldiers in various stages of mental decomposition facing, at least at Madigan Army Medical Center, a compensation review board so hostile that it rewrites the diagnoses of licensed psychiatrists and psychologists, simply to deny benefits to otherwise eligible veterans with shamelessly outspoken justification of saving Army money. It is a scandal beyond all measure, and it will only get worse unless those charged with legal authority take drastic steps to remedy the situation. Simple closure of the forensic unit at Madigan Army Medical Center kicks the inflammatory can down the road to ameliorate political and press inquiries, but it solves nothing.

Even now, new claims from Vietnam veterans for healthcare or disability are coming in to the Department of Veteran Affairs. As both Army suicide expert Colonel Elspeth Ritchie and Mathew Friedman, director of National PTSD Center at Dartmouth, advise, with inattention to the "invisible" wounds of today's wars, hundreds of thousands of new cases will roll into the claims queue for DVA services for years to come.

Even though we speak of PTSD now as a treatable mental illness, in prior wars, we did not. These invisible wounds, wounds to the mind, did not even have an official DSM diagnosis in all wars past; thus there was no issue of compensation payments for them.

As this nation moves towards the fiscal cliff, federal budgets are going to come under the axe, and both the Secretary of Health for the Department of Defense and the Cabinet Secretary of the Department of Veterans Affairs will be no exceptions when lobbyists from the military industrial complex go for the jugular to get their share of the treasury gold.

Although our land wars will ostensibly end by the beginning of 2015—assuming that we don't get into another one in the next couple of years—the costs for these current wars will continue to mount as we pay disability claims, pensions, and medical care for our veterans. And the rear guard now preparing our exodus from Afghanistan will be among the worst hit in the history of U.S. combat psychiatry. We must deal with this now, and deal with it properly.

As we have shown, the main health and long-term disability costs of this war are for enduring injuries to the brain, whether in form of extreme stress or post-concussion syndrome from blasts. These patients and their families are the most disenfranchised and fragmented constituency, seeking an increasingly small portion of table scraps from a dinner table long since vacated. So, rhetoric and principles aside, combat veterans of the War on Terror, as well as millions from other wars, will get less and less of a diminishing share of the budget paid out to the military industrial complex—which not only includes the Boeings and Lockheeds of this nation, as well as foreign militaries, but pension and healthcare benefits administered by Department of Defense and Veterans Affairs. They are in the ring with these known fighters for the military dollar, but they are lightweights. Under our current system, when stacked up against our defense contractors and outsource obligations, the sad truth is that services for our veterans take second place.

The Alliance for Mental Health, a public interest group, advocates awarding Purple Hearts for Post-Traumatic Stress Disorder to force the Department of Defense to take responsibility for what really are their wards—these wounded warriors—to be both contractually and medically made whole before being foisted off into the public safety and health systems, where they will gradually decompose absent the requisite treatment. In other words, whatever we do next, we first have to recognize that the nature of the wars we fight and the stress we put on an undersized military to fight these wars has inflicted wounds that may not bleed on the outside, but internally hemorrhage emotional toxins that distort perception, behavior, and reactions. These toxins rob sufferers of resiliency, their ability to cope, and their ability to navigate in any social setting. Ultimately, these wounds can drive sufferers to kill themselves and others. At the outset, we need to recognize these as war wounds and not a sign of weakness, and it has to be a top-down recognition with penalties for those in command who don't recognize it. Although well meaning for the Alliance for Mental Health to advocate forcing the military to award the Purple Heart to "invisible wounds to the brain" of wounded warriors, it simply is not going to happen, at least not for this cohort of nearly three million combat veterans returning home through 2015.

The outgoing Secretary of Defense Robert Gates, speaking to troops at Forward Operating Base Walton in Kandahar, Afghanistan, on June 7, 2011, said that pensions and healthcare costs are eating the U.S. military alive, and there is no end in sight to escalating costs threatening force protection and national security alike. He's talking about something a whole lot of people don't want to hear about: the rising costs of military health and pension benefits. Neither the military nor General Motors set out to be a healthcare and long-term disability insurers, but after a century of war, that's exactly where the military is. There is no doubt that healthcare and disability costs will consume large portions of the military budget over the next twenty to fifty years. The current solution seems to be to dump the problem onto the public health and safety systems, whose hospitals, jails, prisons, and courts are already overwhelmed with the spewing out of deinstitutionalized, mentally ill civilians. These civilians, many of whom veterans separated from the military, were once wards of the states, but the public health services they consume will inevitably be swamped by a new wave of sick combat veterans simply ushered to the gates of their garrisons—and a huge number will simply get a handshake and, "Thanks for your service. Now go find a job." There were no victory parades for Vietnam veterans, but they at least got a steak dinner and a bus ticket back home, instead of an escort to the garrison gate with a general discharge under honorable conditions, meaning a breach of enlistment contract for disciplinary reasons called "chaptering out"—or, worse, a bed in a nearby homeless shelter.

Half of the nearly three million combat veterans of the War on Terror can be expected to file for long-term disability compensation. This is an unprecedented contractual burden for which neither the Department of Defense nor Department of Veteran Aaffairs are prepared. It is time to face the facts. More than a small percentage of combat veterans are disabled because of combat, particularly with the intensity, "tempo," and multiple deployments of this war. These new veterans have different types of injuries than previous veterans did. That's partly because improvised explosive devices (IEDs) have been the main weapon, and because body armor and improved battlefield trauma care allowed many of them to survive extreme wounds to body and limb that in past wars proved fatal. The VA's medical rehabilitation chief, Dr. David Cifu, said that soldiers are being kept alive at "unprecedented rates." More than 95 percent of troops wounded in Iraq and Afghanistan have survived their visible wounds. However, the invisible wounds far outnumber the visible wounds, and the causality of invisible wounds is a topic still hotly debated in medical and scientific circles.

Most medical and psychology professionals agree that the relentlessness of our Middle Eastern wars and the lack of respite from 24/7 vigilance is one of the causes of invisible psychiatric wounds. Increasingly, a soldier cannot even find a safe place to sleep without a trusted buddy guard awake at bedside, due to infiltration of the ranks of our Afghan ally by the Taliban and sympathizers. Constant, intimate danger has never been a part of warfare for this nation, and Secretary of Defense, Leon Panetta, said that the most frustrating problem of his office was the escalating suicide rate. Operation Enduring Freedom is increasingly a suicide operation that has no realistically accomplishable goals, other than as a political cover for strategic and tactical failures that could cost an election. Bin Laden, who led the attack that set off this War on Terror, was killed a long time ago. Now what? Provide training for the Afghan National Army and local and national police forces? These are the very institutions that the Taliban is infiltrating and publicly bragging about. These are the personnel who are turning their guns on our troops in "green versus blue" shootings. We're exposing our young men and women to the rifle barrels and homemade bombs of the people we're training, who don't want us there and are killing us in increasing numbers. And we wonder why the Army suicide rate is one per day? No one in positions of leadership or command has anything to say about that, other than lower-ranking "yes men" from Central Command, who keep assuring the American public that statistically, we're okay. It's not okay. What's happening in Afghanistan every day is one of the major causes of invisible wounds.

It is no secret that the VA's outmoded system can't keep up with the backlog of claims from the War on Terror, along with the legacy of disabled from wars past, now getting old and demanding their entitlement to free care. More than 1 million veterans currently have delayed disability claims that are more than 300 days old. And as the volume continues to grow and the cost of healthcare for veterans increases, Harvard economist Linda Bilmes estimates that the healthcare and disability costs of the recent wars will cost the nation $600 billion to $900 billion. Despite the mounting claims, Brigadier

General Allison Hickey (USAF ret.), the VA's undersecretary for benefits, has said that the VA is streamlining its process to more effectively take care of veterans, because its mission is to satisfy the needs of the veteran population. She has reiterated that it is important for the Veterans Administration to satisfy the entitlement benefits that veterans should receive as a result of their service.

But how do we take care of that population? How do we handle the million or so disability-eligible returning vets?

Here's how. The President needs to appoint a special paymaster, whether inside or outside the DVA—call it the "Paymaster General"— as he did for the British Petroleum oil spill. That paymaster general will be responsible for getting a "fair and adequate" amount of money into all combat veterans' hands at the time of discharge, so that they have something to help them establish traction as they reenter civilian life and need health care and rehabilitation services. There will be egregious disciplinary problems that are exceptions, but they are relatively few when the flawed Traumatic Brain Injury and behavioral health systems stop doing disability exams and concentrate on diagnosing and treating wounded warriors. Right now the disability determinations are arduous, compromised by faulty information, and even corrupted by claimant and adjudicator alike. We know, however, that exposure to combat is as good an index for predicting future pychiatric disability as any, and there are battlefield reports for every combat exposure—or should be— despite "tempo" of this war. Confronting claimant soldiers with skepticism regarding their traumatic experiences in war may catch 1 percent who are manipulating the system to get undeserved benefits, but is it worth catching the 1 percent at the expense of causing second injury to 99 percent really needing health and rehabilitation services now? In addition, that second injury jacks up the cost of both direct and indirect healthcare costs for the taxpayers—whether through Department of Veterans Affairs claims adjudication; the new Affordable Care Act; municipal, state, and federal departments of corrections, or Social Security Disability Insurance—for complications of untreated PTSD, often evolving into drug and alcohol dependence with associated criminality or psychosomatic diseases like premature coronary artery disease. Thus, even on a cost/benefit basis, it's worth letting the 1 percent slip through, because of the costs associated with misdiagnosing the 99 percent. One way or the other, the United States taxpayer will pick up the direct and indirect healthcare costs for soldiers denied care by the federal government.

How do we incorporate the battlefield records we now have into a paymaster general system of administering immediate benefits and assessing disability claims? With a point system based on the metrics of combat exposure. Specifically, we can assess the number of deployments and number of days under fire, and using these numbers, formulate a fair and equitable metric for brain trauma, whether the Axis IV assessment of severity of stress in DSM IV, post-concussion syndrome on Axis III, or a combination. Most of these cases, but not all, will be blast injuries, but all the cases will be fairly and objectively evaluated. Indeed, there is a percentage of combat vets who will be paid more than they have coming, because for some reason, they are more resilient to psychological trauma. And there will be malingerers stealing from the taxpayers, estimated to be 1 percent of claimants. The vast majority of claimants, however, need significant financial help, and they need it now—not next year, and certainly not in ten. Furthermore, most malingerers can be caught later and dealt with through either civil or criminal legal channels.

With such rapid payments based on a far simpler assessment of potential near- and long-term disability, garrison bases will be cleared of high maintenance and at-risk soldiers, who can be managed and treated in the civilian healthcare system of their communities, as most are anyways. This simply makes fair de jure what is already very unfair de facto; the dumping of sick and at-risk soldiers onto civilian streets to make it or break it on their own. Regardless of whether the Madigan scandal was a variance within the system or the whole system smells, duration of untreated illnesses will decrease, promising better outcomes with lower direct and indirect healthcare costs to the U.S. taxpayer. All that the forensic unit, variance within the system or not, was doing was cost shifting, the technical healthcare jargon for making somebody else pay more for the same illness, just like employees now paying higher co-pays for their healthcare services.

There are certainly obvious exceptions of soldiers needing long-term, specialized care within the military, such as victims of chemical warfare, or in the case of Special Operations, highly classified missions that cannot be disclosed to even a private physician. But again, this unique population is not the one causing the problem. Although medical and socially complex, it is relatively small in numbers. For the rest, they need to go home with assistance in connecting to a primary care provider who has access to meaningful military healthcare records from deployments to get returning vets into effective clinical pathways for their medical care and rehabilitation, informed by valid diagnostics.

The Urgency of Addressing Veteran Affairs

Now, except for blips in the news with headlines of a bad incident involving a veteran, very little is said about veteran affairs in the political arena. There are no Congressional districts to be determined in an election by advocating for combat veterans and the trillions of dollars to take care of them. Senator Patty Murray may raise the red flag about medical care, but few have heard her. However, our veterans are coming home and entering civilian life. The ripples of their return are being felt from small towns in rural America to the L.A. suburbs. As the adjustment from military to civilian life begins en masse, the public is not as blind or confounded as politicians make them out to be. Most people either have a vet in the family or know one. And most people know what the vets have to go through in order to have a new beginning in civilian life, medically as well as fiscally. Where at the infinite line of claims adjustors are Department of Veterans Affairs psychiatrists and neurologists for their Post-Traumatic Stress Disorder and Traumatic Brain Injuries, respectively? Where is the health care, and where are the jobs?

The public is very disturbed by this serious social problem, and politicians and officials alike simply confuse them more. So, instead of haggling like medical insurance adjusters, we need to get the money into the veterans' hands, then build out the medical infrastructure before hiring any more adjudicators and claims adjusters. Treat the medical problems first, facilitate the reintegration of veterans into civilian life with all the services the VA can muster, push Congress to pass a jobs bill for veterans by offering accelerated tax credits to businesses that hire them, provide aggressive job training and education opportunities for veterans, and expand emergency medical care to encompass civilian hospitals as well as veteran hospital facilities. Access to medical care and rehabilitation when needed— rather than after adjudicated by claims adjustors—will cut down on long-term disability by reducing duration of untreated illnesses, thus preventing progression of stress and traumatic brain syndromes into more serious problems, whether they are medical complications, like heart disease, or violence and suicides.

Long-Term Disability

The Department of Veterans Affairs and the military alike need to get out of the long-term disability business, which reeks of corruption, inefficiency, and bad faith because counter-insurgency warfare is an uninsurable risk. At least that is what for-profit insurance company underwriters have concluded. This one-million-man-march of disabled veterans coming home is no less a disaster than Katrina, September 11th itself, and the BP oil spill. Therefore, treat it as such a one-off event and get the doctors in these VA and military hospitals back to treating the wounded and dedicating themselves to their mission of force health protection, not making them doctors who are made to think like insurance doctors or disability claims managers. Insurance doctors are a different breed of medical graduate, because they are adversarial to the patient. They belong in insurance companies and not anywhere near military hospitals. That was the lesson of the Joint Base Lewis-McChord scandal at Madigan Army Medical Center, which the Army's Surgeon General described as a "variance" from the norm of assessing medical claims. The "variance" General Horoho talked about should be zero. No more blind spots for isolated weed patches of forensic units to sprout. No variance systemically within the system either.

Fitness-for-Duty

Fitness-for-duty examinations should be the same as annual flight physicals for pilots. The purpose of fitness-for-duty examination should not be to determine whether a combat veteran is a "bad soldier" and undeserving of compensation or later support for neuropsychiatric disability showing up months or years later. It should be to rate the soldier accurately on the military's Electronic Health Record The Fitness for Duty (FFD) profile is there to be updated and maintained with every clinical encounter to show every soldier's current state of health – or fitness for duty. Here is the rating mnemonic currently embedded in the Army Electronic Health Record:

P – General physical condition, stamina, or any problem not addressed below.

U – Upper extremities and upper (cervical and thoracic) spine.

L – Lower extremities and lower (lumbosacral) spine.

H – Hearing and ear conditions.

E – Eyesight and eye conditions.

S – Psychiatric conditions.

How many soldiers are being deployed without accurate and regularly updated fitness-for-duty profiles? It is doubtful that Sergeant Bales had a thorough fitness-for-duty profile entered into AHLTA before his last deployment. If he did, it would have required a waiver from the base commander for him to be fit for duty. Such a waiver has not been reported in his case. Again, this profiling module for fitness-for-duty currently embedded in the Army's Electronic Health Record can either capture vicissitudes of long-term disability through cycles of deployments or fail its function of maintaining Force Health Protection through sloppy maintenance. Can you kick a soldier out without benefits if he is rated as impaired from the psychological and neuropsychiatric complications of a blast injury on the "S" rating of "PULHES" module in the Army's Electronic Health Record?

To say this is not an issue in the military is simply denial. Commanders and doctors alike, who are determined to chapter a soldier out without benefits, thence to be filtered through the public safety net, do not want impairment on S. It is therefore not the focus of military doctors' attention, particularly psychiatrists and clinical psychologists.

Fitness-for-duty examinations should have one purpose: to determine whether the soldier can fight another day or not, and if not, to ascertain whether treatment of any type can restore him/her to fighting capability. This does not take an experienced military psychiatrist or clinical psychologist many hours to determine. The reason for so much time being spent per soldier is to document thoroughly a compensable presentation requiring a Medical Evaluation Board for long-term disability or justify chaptering him out to get in the long line for VA claims adjudication. Personnel overhead for direct costs of military healthcare should not be spent on either protecting oneself from the Monday morning quarterbacking of reviewers, like the forensic unit at Madigan, where medical diagnoses were arbitrarily altered or to assist in appropriate disciplinary actions without medicalizing all aberrant behavior, thus undermining necessary hierarchical command for war.

Commanders need to keep discipline in their units and cannot be controlled by the medicalization of every violation of regulations. Such medicalization, when unwarranted, does undermine discipline. But medical determinations take an hour, not many hours or days. Now, military psychiatrists are too bogged down in fitness-for-duty exams because they are the point of the spear leading to medical evaluation boards that set the stage for costly and life-changing long-term disability payments; they are vulnerable, therefore, lending medical legitimacy to minimizing the number of compensable diagnoses that we cited in the Madigan scandal. If things were changed, and military psychiatry and clinical psychology had no role in determining long-term disability, more accurate, consistent, and valid fitness-for-duty profiling would occur, thereby enhancing force health protection, the primary duty of military medicine. And, as cited above, the receiving primary care doctor taking responsibility for the veteran after discharge will have the beginning of an accurate roadmap—called clinical pathway—on which to proceed in the veteran's lifetime care.

If the soldier can be returned to duty with treatment, then the most effective treatment trial should be provided. It is the rare FFD exam where this is a very complex matter. Either the soldier is motivated to fight another day if treated or not treated. Rarely is this motivation hard to determine. One experienced military psychiatrist simply asks every hospitalized psychiatric patient on active duty whether he/she wants to stay in the army. The answer is rarely ambiguous. So, whether it's a non-compensable character flaw or it's a compensable neuropsychiatric disorder, get the ones who have no intention of fighting another day off the base and back home with proper care plans and accurate clinical documentation for case managers and primary care providers in their communities.

Military and VA Healthcare Changes

All of this sounds like a costly restructuring of military and DVA healthcare. Like any restructuring, there will be a first-time charge for such drastic changes to a system operationally structured for another era and other wars of the past when neuropsychiatric disability was not obstructing the care and dispositions for veterans. PTSD was not a diagnosis in prior wars with such a large number of returning combat veterans, and TBIs were not such a large issue as they are now, although they certainly did occur and were considered minor head injuries. Not even sports medicine practitioners believe that anymore, although until recently they did.

Military and DVA healthcare should not be geared for the next large-scale land war, because we probably won't have one. We know it is unlikely to have thousands of boots on the ground as strangers in faraway places. Robert Gates told us so, and Vice President Biden said we're not going to write any more checks for that. National security may mean that the Mexican border is of more importance to U.S. security than that of the northwest territories of Pakistan and Afghanistan. And the warming of the Arctic Ocean is bringing foreign flags to a once-frozen sea, much to the consternation of the U.S. Navy. Canada will require support in defense of its Arctic territorial waters, as will we in Alaska. And how will the Army Engineers get water to drought-stricken parts of the continental United States if we still want to keep our nation's breadbasket irrigated? What will we do when our allies fight amongst themselves over water and diminishing natural resources? These are just examples of what our Pentagon war planners are now gaming on their computers, as opposed to a massive ground invasion of Syria or Iran.

Our military is simply not big enough as it is currently structured and financed to handle a large-scale land war. The draft was such a failure for Vietnam that it was not even considered on September 12, 2001. And the contemptuous attitude towards the current returning combat veteran with the recurrent dumping of sick and at-risk soldiers into communities by essentially mistaking breach of recruitment contract for felony charges, is all but a declaration of failure of an all-volunteer army that still requires the National Guard to support its rear guard action in Afghanistan. Our recommendations can only work if the urgency of President Eisenhower's encomium for the citizen-soldier is finally taken seriously.

The draft was discriminatory and was disastrous in Vietnam, but the recruitment and recurrent breaches of contract, whether active or passive, in the all-volunteer army is equally discriminatory and approaching the same—or possibly worse—proportions of the Vietnam draft. Mercenary armies, private contract armies, and an all-volunteer force supported by undertrained and underarmed National Guard units simply don't work. We see that in Afghanistan through the eyes of our own mass media. In order to improve military healthcare and find the appropriate system for addressing invisible wounds that invariably occur when there is inequality in military service requires great political courage to effect a dramatic change in the concept of national service.

Universal Military Training

The epidemic of violence like the acts of Stewart, Stroh, Dorner, and Bales are like dense red mercury rising. Similarly, the epidemic of suicides cannot seem to be controlled. These tragedies occur, in part, because of the inequities in military service. Our army of volunteers is overstressed, overtaxed, and overdeployed, but under-maintained. Put simply, we need more boots on the ground, here and wherever our military is deployed. Universal military training, as horrific as it sounded forty years ago, gets rid of both of these inequities in military service. The poor kid drafted out of an urban low-income working neighborhood for Vietnam and the poor country boy sold on a patriotic means to better himself both joined the Army, while children of the one-percenters went to Europe or continued their educations and let their disadvantaged avatars take their places. It was unfair and politically unsustainable. The solution to form an all-volunteer military was equally unsuccessful, because the inequities still exist. Let's erase them.

With UMT, everyone enters basic training upon completion of high school, or agrees to enter for two years following completion of a specialized education necessary for the military—specifically something like the Barry Plan allowing doctors to complete specialty training before entering the military as general medical officers. But everyone, male and female, goes for a year of training, followed by recurrent training as either active reservists or guardsmen. A high school diploma is a requirement for basic training. No diploma? Welcome to summer school for a six-month GED course tacked onto your service obligation. Need remediation in language and math skills? You can start on Sesame Street for phonics, but everyone sits for and passes a GED exam, even if it means a regimen of English as a Second Language courses. Conscientious objectors can be recognized, but they will serve two years in the Peace Corps, Job Corps, Head Start, or equivalent volunteer group, or take on EMT training and serve as medics or community paramedics. And just as President Eisenhower suggested, there is room for dramatic physical or mental impairment deferments.

Through a national service universal military training requirement, just like the Israelis have, the whole issue of entitlements for special sacrifices gets erased. When the war in Afghanistan is over, Operation Enduring Freedom will no longer be a military operation demanding large-scale deployments of troops and equipment to build new regimes on foreign soil. Our responsibility is to our own homeland, and homeland security is every citizen's responsibility. That means that every citizen should expect to take on the big community or national service, whether helping Mayor Emmanuel neutralize street gangs in Chicago, clean up Zucotti Park after the latest round of sleep-in demonstrations, or serve on a destroyer in the Persian Gulf. This is true equality in obligation of service. And the benefits that will flow therefrom will enable those discharged at the completion of their national service for low-interest education loans, specialized grants, job training, and a form of single-payer national health insurance. The Departments of Defense and Veterans Affairs would soon no longer have any responsibility for determining whether a soldier or veteran is really disabled from combat or scamming the system. Their missions will be clear: treating the injuries of war and military service, not running disability insurance companies. It is simply beyond the capacity of our Departments of Defense and Veterans Affairs, despite rhetorical promises to improve services. They are so far behind the curve due to lack of preparedness for this war that they can not catch up. The money and resources simply are not there, nor will they ever be.

Military Discharge

Once a soldier is discharged due to being no longer fit for duty and has enough money to establish him/herself at home, then there should be streamlined Supplemental Security Income court for all War on Terror soldiers not already compensated for their service or disabilities. If invisible wounds of war emerge later on, the veterans will know where to go because of special Supplemental Security Income hearing processes that are streamlined and informed of veterans' disabilities. This is already happening in the form of veterans courts for criminal issues. How else are the hundreds of thousands of veterans now without any benefits—whether pawning their medals to survive, too sick to even make it inside a shelter, or too addicted, impulsive, or too distorted with rage to stay out of prison—eating? This is not a small number of outliers. It is a disgraceful number in the hundreds of thousands for which the Departments of Defense and Veterans Affairs have no legitimate excuses, as these sick veterans are really wards of the federal government. But the federal government doesn't want them. Enlistment contracts are being breached, with too many appeals being made to make them right. Therefore, let's not try to fix a system that cannot be fixed. Let's replace it with a discharge mechanism that works.

Transforming the Veterans Administration

Some will say, as has been said, "You can't just blow up the VA." There are too many disabled veterans from too many wars both dependent upon and very satisfied with the care they receive at the

VA. This should not be stopped. Our recommendations are for the future, not retroactive. In this scenario, the Department of Veterans Affairs continues on, but it is out of the long-term disability insurance business that has drawn it such flak, diverted its resources, and too often corrupted it. There are no headline complaints about veterans already inside the tent and receiving care. Certainly some care is great, and some not so great. But that is not the problem. DVA is the gateway for the support of this all-volunteer army personnel being discharged, both with some benefits and without any, into civilian society. It can no longer be effective as a gateway that operates for a past era. It needs to transform for the future. With specialized Supplemental Security Income hearing processes under the Department of Health and Human Services, and universal healthcare now the law of the land, it can narrow its focus to managing and protecting our veterans without continuing its role as a supplementary healthcare provider and the largest long-term disability insurance claims management company in the world. That certainly was not the intent of Congress when creating the Veterans Administration.

We advocate for making good on the recruitment contracts made with the all-volunteer army, whether regulars, guardsmen, or active reservists. We also expect all contracts between DVA and current employees and outside vendors be maintained. With time, of course, DVA will become smaller. Claims administrators will have plenty of opportunities working in the Supplemental Security Income hearing system (SSI), where long-term disability assessments will have to be made, just as they do now with SSI. But they cannot simply deny half the claims in the first round of SSI claims, as is now the practice, and force the sick and disabled into hearings processes to save money in a war of attrition, again promising more to the public than can possibly be paid out. This book is not about either healthcare reform, entitlement systems, or their implementation and management in some vague future or past. It is about the invisible wounds of war and how they affect military discharges, and how we can improve the system.

There is already a built-in path to efficient reform of the DVA system. Specialized SSI courts need to get up to speed—a sort of legal reform—to work efficiently, professionally, and fairly. There will be plenty of opportunities for DVA claims personnel wishing to continue on with this type of work by transferring to the SSI process. And, on the healthcare side of DVA, clinicians may wish to carry on with their special work with this special patient populations, or follow this new generation of veterans into community practice—whether private practice, nursing home, rehab facilities, substance abuse clinics, head injury programs, or specialized traumatic stress disorders programs. Finally, as demands for services from the DVA gradually decrease, certainly valuable assets will become surplused. They should be sold off, with the proceeds being cycled only one direction: into a special trust fund to pay for this DVA restructuring and to put money into the pockets of soldiers before—not after—they return home broke and jobless. Veterans will need the highest quality of benefit guarantees, not the cheapest that turns away community providers because of lack of funding, as is currently the case. That means traditional medical insurers must have the same respect of clinicians in private practice as do other high-quality insurers. That means insurerers must be capitalized, as well as government-friendly carriers like United Healthcare.

Social Security hearing processes will need to be funded. The monies will come from eliminating DVA and DOD disability claims determinations and processing. Ultimately, disability funding for veterans will have to come from the Social Security mechanism rather than from the DVA disability and healthcare processes. The Social Security Administration can provide a more streamlined force health service in the military and a reduced demand for healthcare services from the DVA, which are so backlogged with claims that veterans have to wait for over a year and a half just to get their claims heard. And it will only get worse by January, 2015.

The Electronic Health Record

All military computer-based medical records and clinical evaluation systems, from ordering consultations to keeping track of each soldier's medical history, should be completely compatible with each other as if they were on a single cloud-storage distributed database computer system. The once-hyped Wounded Warrior Program, designed to track the cycle of all wounds from initial care to either death or return to duty, is a brilliant idea made possible by the capabilities of AHLTA and its counterpart, the electronic health recor of the DVA, known as VISTA (Veterans Health Information Systems and Technology Architecture). The battles, squabbling, and inexcusable waste expended on intelligent software development to enable this worthy cause of the interoperability and data management of military health records is scandalous. As one Canadian trauma surgeon recently returned from NATO assignment in Afghanistan said, "I had to work at Kandahar, and the military EHR—presumably CHCS I— was in DOS." In other words, the system of health records was built on an antiquated computer operating system from the 1980s. CHCS I is designed primarily for ordering consultations, but what good is it if a neurologist cannot get a psychiatrist to evaluate a traumatic brain injury patient because the psychiatrists are being deployed elsewhere? The computer designed to arrange for a consult cannot find a consulting physician because that physician is not reachable by the electronic system designed to reach him or her. The delay in getting that consult is unacceptable, especially when the system implemented to provide for that consult doesn't work. Therefore, what good is it if ordering clinical psychological evaluation on a complex fitness-for-duty exam simply does not go through in a timely fashion, so that the disturbed soldier ends up in the brig? None of these multiple service clinical IT systems, as expensive to the taxpayers and burdensome to clinicians as they are, can even talk to each other. That, too, is unacceptable. We are promised that this will be fixed by 2014 with a new DOD contractor, anticipating the enabling of AHLTA, CHCSI, Essentris, Navy Systems, Air Force Systems, and DVA VISTA to talk to each other. We shall see, but already DOD and DVA have said they will not develop a combined system as promised. Again, millions will be spent on the margins with only the hope and prayer of some miraculous technical innovation still nowhere in sight, despite promises of the Wounded Warrior Program (AW2) to track wounds from their earliest field treatment to either total remission or death.

Barring a black swan event, such as Syria's deployment of chemical/biological weapons, there should be no major ground actions overseas, which means that the pressure should be off the military in terms of processing wounded personnel on a large scale. Therefore, the military should have some breathing room to integrate medical record-keeping systems. The question is, how to do it efficiently? Few would dispute that VISTA is better than AHLTA. So why spend millions on upgrading AHLTA? Why not make VISTA the electronic health record for all services, including DVA? Arguments that each service has its own special needs that DVA cannot address is simply specious, and one more example of interservice and interagency rivalries that the public is sick of paying for.

The president, as commander-in-chief, has the authority and could order all services to switch DOD and DVA clinical record keeping to VISTA at his next cabinet meeting, but that's a rat's nest of special interests, both inside and outside the Department of Defense. First Epic, a company from Madison, Wisconsin, was to get the contract to make all these systems interoperable. Now it is Harris Corporation. Why the change? Is it relevant? It certainly is, if we are truly seeking the best clinical IT for wounded warriors. And it certainly is when billions have already been spent for this seemingly impossible enterprise software project, and more is about to be spent. So where should the cash come from for this one-off payment to returning vets? Start by scrapping AHLTA and making VISTA the electronic health records system for all services and the Department of Veterans Affairs. It is reputedly one of the best electronic health records system, and it has the interoperability already that DOD has not been able to attain.

It has just been publicized that, after burning through $1 billion of $5 billion for merging DOD and DVA healthcare IT, nothing was accomplished and all efforts to do so have terminated. It would cost, they say, $12 billion. Many experts have expressed conviction that, instead of seeking interoperability across multiple platforms, best simply go with VISTA. In other words, billions have been spent since the Surgeon General told us by email in 2008 that AHLTA is the main reason for clinical professionals leaving services, but nothing has been accomplished. Why? Imagine were it Oracle making this announcement, after blowing billions! Or, Mayo Clinic, heavily dependent on federal financing of its EHR via Medicare! But, it is just the military again, probably paying hundreds for toilet seats, the public probably figures. Oh well, just one big yawn. Next announcement?

Chapter 11

Solutions and Benefits

We've covered the basic moral and administrative issues in play as our soldiers return home. Insofar as immediate medical solutions are concerned, first, the entire diagnosis from emergency triage through the life cycle of the invisible wounds of war must be addressed. This requires embedding at least rudimentary artificial intelligence into an integrated Electronic Health Record platform in order to bring discipline to all clinicians entering their opinions and judgments of "problems" into a soldier and veteran's clinical history. Especially for the signature injury of the war on terror and its nearly 3,000,000 combat veterans, the electronic health records should be integrated into a robust, portable, and combined telepsychiatry and teleneurology system, complete with state-of-art on-time neuroimaging. This is a system that should walk clinicians through intake sluice gates that are fail-safe for identifying so-called invisible wounds of war that heighten risk of lethal outcomes. Such lethal outcomes include suicides and violence, as well as deterioration into chronic psychiatric and psychosomatic disorders

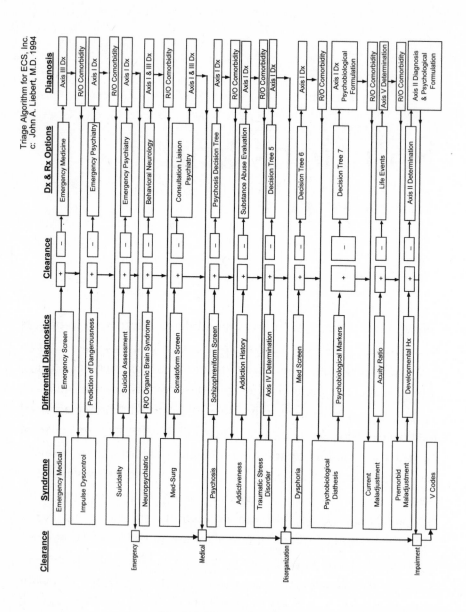

Triage Algorithm for ECS, Inc.
c: John A. Liebert, M.D. 1994

The JAL Triage Algorithm

caused by extended durations of untreated Post-Traumatic Stress Disorder, Traumatic Brain Injuries, and other psychiatric disorders. Additionally, with the global war on terror, they include occult medical/surgical diseases with higher likelihood of occurrence in a population of young men and women returning—or returned—from multiple combat deployments in far-off lands. These soldiers do acquire exotic parasitic diseases not acquired at home; clinicians must be alert to the exigencies demanded of such infections not on diagnostic radar screens in the United States.

There are many Computerized Clinical Decision Support Systems (CDSS) available for this task, but the "JAL Triage Algorithm©" serves as an example of one that incorporates defaults for ruling out medical/surgical diseases and psychiatric disorders based on severity of time-determined need for clinical intervention and likelihood of presentation at any given point of entry, whether Bishkek AFB, Kyrgizstan or Fort Bragg, North Carolina.

As seen, an Electronic Health Record with such an embedded CDSS algorithm demands that the clinician assesses the patient methodically—rather than arbitrarily responding to a symptom set, such as insomnia and low back pain—by naming the problems and then prescribing for them as follows:

"Problem 1, Insomnia – Treatment, Ambien"
"Problem 2, Low Back Pain – Treatment, Vicodin"

It is known that all clinicians have a need for more information every day of their practice than they can call up from memory or learning. So, such symptomatic diagnoses and treatments like this are more often than not going to miss the mark. Why, for example, is the patient not sleeping? And, what will a powerful narcotic do for the potential of emotional numbing—or need to numb—from PTSD, as well as ultimate relief of disability and suffering from low back pain? This is an extreme example of bad practices, only cited here for purposes of demonstrating the need for more diagnostic discipline across the system for returning and returned soldiers—as well as new deployments.

These soldiers have weapons, will have them wherever they go, and know how to use them in hair-trigger response to perceived threat. How could fired LAPD officer Christopher Dorner have been picked up as a psychiatric inpatient so he would not have been alone in his pickup truck with a loaded firearm at his side? Despite the pronouncements from former police chiefs and retired criminal-profilers-turned-television-pundits, when Dorner's training officer did not get this man into a reintegration program after he broke down in tears in a patrol car, it was a moment of prevention that was lost. And five people are now dead because that opportunity was lost.

By integrating the analytics of clinical decision-making into AHLTA, clinicians could be limited in entering diagnoses in the problem list; criteria for diagnosis, as cited by Paul Miller, would have to be fully investigated with the patient and either ruled in or out. Entering "Depression NOS," for example, informs clinicians of almost nothing, as was the case when Cho Seung-hui was discharged back to the Virginia Tech campus after brief involuntary detention in the local hospital with the diagnosis of Depression NOS. "Not Otherwise Specified" means that he could have been depressed for any reason, not necessarily having to do with any psychosis. He could have been reentering his cohort of a large population of college students on a Sunday afternoon, who were simply depressed for reasons not otherwise specified, such as a hangover, facing consequences of procrastinating in preparation of paper to be handed in the following morning, the downer after "the party's over," a bad date, no date, or other unspecified reasons. In other words, Depression NOS is more often than not, as in the case of Cho Seung-hui's involuntary detention evaluation for suicide and dangerousness, useless. How can such a vast landscape of problem entries be removed from the pure judgment decried by Miller in his pursuit of Computer Assisted Diagnostic Interview (CADI), demanding assessment of criteria as signs and symptoms of a disorder—rather than intuitive jumping to conclusions, rightly or wrongly, strictly based on experience and clinical judgment? Clinicians are human and subject to being subjective, and can even be prejudiced about their patients.

Medication Interactions and Contra-indications

When prescribing a medication on AHLTA, the prescriber cannot submit any drug to the pharmacist until he or she reviews potential interactions with drugs patient currently takes and potential adverse reactions of the drug, and then decides to push the "override" button. This forces the clinician to at least think about prescribing a drug that could increase the metabolic destruction of another critical drug, possibly impairing the treatment efforts of another physician. For example, Prozac, on top of certain cancer drugs, will reduce the blood levels of some chemotherapy, and therefore increase the risk of a cancer patient's early demise. Such discipline should be built into AHLTA for reducing the risk of missing potentially lethal mental states of unremitting human destructiveness, too.

Certainly, no clinicians can predict violent acts to self, others, or both with 100 percent certainty and must respect the patient's rights. But this is today's Army, with an epidemic of suicides and way too many murders and assaults. Therefore, there must be collateral discipline in the methodical discipline of searching for risk factors of suicides and violence when the uncommon opportunity of interviewing a soldier presents itself. There is no substitute for face-to-face clinical interviews by competent and experienced clinicians if the current epidemic of suicides is to be stopped. It can be done, but it will require as clinically intelligent computer development for AHLTA as was described for e-prescribing, that is, a prompt or voice prompt saying, "Doctor, you said patient has insomnia and low back pain. Is he depressed? Please document that the following risk factors for suicide have either been ruled out or verified." Such software analytics require an algorithm, such as the JAL Triage Algorithm. With the JAL Triage Algorithm©, one can see that the examining clinician must clear "Emergency" before simply closing out and discharging the patient into the community with potentially lethal outcome.

Of course, medical emergencies must be ruled out. You recall the case of Sergeant J, returning on compassionate leave from MP duty in Saigon after Tet and collapsing on the psychiatrist's floor. Medical emergencies come first, but then the clinician needs to make certain the patient is not imminently dangerous. When Officer Right quickly drew his weapon to show the psychiatrist how fast things can sour on the street, the psychiatrist not only got a lesson about being a cop, but he knew immediately that his own life was in danger. There can be no weapons in the clinical space. Clinicians have been murdered in military psychiatric clinics in Iraq during war and at Fairchild AFB, Spokane during peacetime. Just like the FBI Academy at Quantico, no weapons are allowed inside the institution. Weapons are checked in, perhaps serviced, and then checked out when the soldier leaves.

Strange Behavior

If a patient is behaving strangely, as was Cho during his hospitalization, dangerousness must be ruled out first to protect the clinician, the public, and the patient himself.

Illustrations of Strange Behavior, Non Verbal, the Case of Cho Seung-hui

In the case of Cho Seung-hui, Cho described his infestation with mites to a family doctor, who could not find any physical residue of mite infestation. This was a delusion that later turned malignantly lethal because Cho, as he approached the day of his mass murder and his own death, withdrew further and further into his delusions until he was almost in a limbic trance, walking through his own psychotic projection of narcissistic persecution. It was from within that trance state that Cho acted out his own final steps. Only it was real.

A roommate describes Cho's final ritual in preparation for his suicidal mass murder:

"5:00 a.m.: While in Suite 2121 of Harper Hall, Joseph E. 'Joe' Aust, one of Cho's five roommates, noticed that Cho was awake and at his computer.

"Around 5:30 a.m.: Karan Grewal, one of Cho's other roommates, noticed Cho, clad in boxer shorts and a T-shirt, brushing his teeth and applying acne cream.

"Between 5:30 and 6:00 a.m.: Aust saw Cho return from the bathroom, get dressed, and leave.

"Before 7:00 a.m.: Cho was seen waiting outside an entrance to West Ambler Johnston Hall.

"Before 7:15 a.m.: Emily Hilscher was dropped off at her West Ambler Johnston Hall dormitory by her boyfriend, Karl D. Thornhill.

"7:15 a.m.: A 911 emergency call to Virginia Tech campus police reported a shooting at West Ambler Johnston Hall, leaving Ryan Christopher Clark, the resident adviser, dead, and Emily Hilscher fatally wounded in Room 4040, which housed Hilscher."

From there, after preparing his videotape for overnighting to NBC News, Cho took his weapons into Norris Hall, chained the exit doors shut, and began his murder spree. The notation that Cho was depressed "not otherwise specified," for no specific reason, completely missed the point that the depressed and apparently mute student was not depressed at all, even after brandishing a knife the night before and promising to commit suicide. The depressed student suffered from Schizophrenia, and in the midst of a psychotic delusional state, was likely preoccupied with auditory hallucinations, making him mute or preoccupied in a world of voices yelling or talking to him. This is why any computer-assisted diagnostic interview protocol has to permit a line of questioning that does not allow for a blanket lack of specificity regarding a symptom.

The clinician in his encounter with an unknown or unremembered patient has presumably now established as secure frame for examination. To "work smart" in fast-paced clinical settings like ERs and military clinics, the clinician must be "epidemiologically-informed," knowing the "likelihood" of certain presentations of patients at his particular site. The Secretary of Defense has declared an epidemic of suicides in active-duty military personnel. That may be the actual context or framework for the examination. Therefore, the next step is to rule out suicide. Even in civilian practice, this should be a routine default in fast-paced clinical encounters with patients, because research shows that 80 percent of completed suicides were preceded by visits to a primary care provider, with documented desire to discuss suicidal ideation. Cho presented to a private doctor complaining of infestation with mites—obviously a delusion that the doctor should have recognized. The next thing is to rule out dangerousness to the self and others, rather than merely prescribing acne medication. Cho was delusional.

Accordingly, how can busy clinicians, whether in civilian or military practice settings, pick up the actively suicidal person in that rare and singular moment when he presents clinically? The clinician must listen carefully to what the patient says and flag anything that even seems like a suicidal ideation or a desire to cause self-harm. The obvious warnings, which we've covered in detail above, are affirmations of suicidal attempt or intent, prior attempts at suicide, ideations of suicide, dreams of suicide, expressions of hopelessness, unrelenting and unmanageable physical pain, seething anger or hostility towards self or others, statements of crippling guilt, and proximity to any weapons combined with any of the above. Remember two things: People who tell you what they are going to do almost inevitably do it; a suicidal individual has nothing else to lose. These two caveats alone can save lives in a clinical situation, as well as the life of the patient.

Now, assuming the monkey of long-term disability determinations and management is off the back of healthcare providers in the military and VA medical centers, best practices can be 100 percent the mission of clinical services. Forensic units won't be threatening clinicians with what diagnoses they make because of the cost to taxpayers for one diagnosis or another. Chaptering that strips the soldier of post-discharge benefits as an efficient means of getting troubled soldiers out of the army will not be necessary, thus making combat veterans, their families, and our societies safer. There will be three million of them, all but rare ones exposed to combat in multiple deployments. So, assuming the DOD and the DVA—through the channel provided by The Wounded Warrior Program—come up with an effective and interoperable electronic health record that covers the whole enterprise serving soldiers coming in, serving, and leaving the military, improved diagnostics can be expected. And with improved diagnostics, we should expect to see earlier and better treatments for Post-Traumatic Stress Disorder, Traumatic Brain Injuries, substance abuse, violent impulse disorders, and suicidality—especially because doctors will be thinking of two things: reliable diagnosis, advocated by Miller, and valid diagnosis, advocated by Klein. Both of these drive a treatment plan more likely to work, particularly with inevitable handoffs from clinician to clinician, whether remaining in the military or transferring to civilian care at home.

To do this, there needs to be discipline imposed by all clinicians entering both clinical observations and opinions, such as "problems," into the EHR. It should not be enough to shoot from the hip and enter "adjustment disorder" for a soldier who can't sleep, is irritable, and has changing moods. Now, within the political and bureaucratic culture of military medicine, such an entry does not get a clinician in as much trouble as entering Post-Traumatic Stress Disorder; that is the lesson of the Madigan Scandal. Any DOD or DVA official arguing otherwise is either in total denial or a liar.

Today's combat veteran presenting in a TBI, ER, psychiatric inpatient unit, or behavioral health clinic can be very confusing. Clinicians can understand the context of that soldier's service record and home in on a problem the same way Google Earth homes in on the Olympic stadium. One can see that it's in London, but where? Different clues may lead you to different searches and destinations. That's like the initial presentation in presentation-based clinical practice, where different clinicians may agree on a general context for a presentation, but be led down divergent paths by different clues. Absent verifiable agreement on common clues, there is diagnostic chaos that leads nowhere. Too often this is the case in the computer-assisted diagnostic interviews now supported by AHLTA, in which many clinicians looking for the same thing—valid diagnosis of soldier's presenting symptoms that inform effective clinical interventions—without which the patient will either not get well, or get worse and even die.

Such diagnostic validity should be the primary goal of the Wounded Warrior Program clinical IT investment, but it is not. In fact, one can argue that having all multiple diagnostic screeners unreliable in naming the problem in AHLTA actually can save the government millions. One clinician entering Personality Disorder means a pre-existing condition preceding four combat tours that arguably is responsible for all his/her problems might be preferred in the current state of Military and VA Medicine, where clinicians have to worry about diagnosing compensable illnesses that are combat-related with lifetime disability. What, for example, happened to veteran Madigan Psychiatrist, Dr Hicks, who ended up the main loser in the Madigan investigation? Discharge the soldier as easily as possible without the burden of a Medical Evaluation Board Examination and let the VA adjudicators sort it out in about a year. Or, almost equally good is a scatter in which each screener picks a different symptom because each is following a similar but different clue. Like searching on a smartphone navigation program, as you enter each letter, the computer makes a suggestion. Simply deadening your brain to a decision and following the suggestion can lead you to the wrong place. This is what our current electronic records and screening system can do, making it difficult to come up with a differential diagnosis. Such invalid reliability of wrong diagnosis or scatter is the oxygen of the forensic unit that was recently disbanded. Healthcare IT is supposed to fix the problem, but it has not. In fact, arguably, in the case of AHLTA, it has made it worse.

Until the Secretary of Health for the Department of Defense makes diagnostic reliability in the cause of diagnostic validity the priority for the current epidemic of PTSD, TBIs, assaults, and suicides in the military, the system will continue to fall short of its mission. Actually, Dr. Paul Miller did speak to clinical staff at Madigan Army Medical Center about computer-assisted diagnostic interviewing. Unfortunately, it fell on deaf ears. Psychopharmacology experts from the Neuroscience Education Institute, including Dr. Stephen Stahl and his PTSD and TBI experts, met with command at Fort Hood. Likewise, their message of making a valid diagnosis to select evidence-based treatment—as Donald Klein has long advocated—fell on deaf ears. Getting it right diagnostically is simply not what anyone wants to hear in any organization of clinicians vexed by treating patients whose diagnoses may generate millions of dollars of lifetime, long-term disability benefits.

Civilians with the financial means would not tolerate the bad practices that are presently institutionalized within the military and VA systems, but soldiers and their families have no choice. Military command is suffused with ambiguities. Should a returning combat vet who's mentally ill have the same rights to good-faith and first-class treatment as a civilian with resources to pay on a civilian basis? Where, for example, do generals go for their treatment? Do General Powell and Petraeus have to wait in line for help at their local VA and then deal with a bank of military claims adjusters? Rank has its privileges. That goes for health and pensions as much as it does for lots of other things in the military. The lack of equality of service is a serious problem that demands fast repair, or old military and VA processes for past wars will haunt this nation for years to come, possibly worse than the debacle of Vietnam did.

Looking at a New York City subway or D.C. Metro map is like looking at the ER rack that has the neighborhoods of "presentations" for Head Injury, Abdominal Pain, Strange Behavior, Self-Harm, Assault, Limb Problem, Mentally Ill, Intoxicated. All the cases we cited presented with one or more of these clinical presentations. So that is where the clinician starts: entering these presentations as problems into the EHR, AHLTA, or VISTA. As we throw around the term "meaningful use" under the Affordable Care Act, what is meaningful usefulness of another machine to operate in a busy practice if it doesn't have the functionality to discipline the clinician into getting a diagnosis that the next doctor can understand and either agree with or state—"I disagree, because."

Psychiatric Interview

After the "emergency" presentations are ruled in, which can be done by a well-trained medic, the physician can determine how much time she has to work up the patient. A confused man sent from a military ER can be accepted for psychiatric evaluation by a psychologist with no medical training. That patient, then evaluated by the psychologist, may actually be diabetic with hypoglycemia, or very low blood sugar, and thus may present confusion or disorientation, which are symptoms of hypoglycemia. Did anyone run this patient's blood glucose, a fifteen second test? There is no time to work this patient up. He should never have been sent from the ER in the first place, but these things do happen. This confused man does not need a workup for TBI or PTSD, but an injection of glucose for hypoglycemia or a couple of oranges. He comes back to his senses and tells the clinician he hasn't had anything to eat while waiting in the ER and psych clinic. His blood glucose has dropped so low that he is confused, disoriented, and on the verge of insulin shock. So unless the clinician knows the patient well, he must take him as he is and without judgment interfering with the classical rules of triage, and work this patient up as altered mental status. That requires Throwing out the WWHHHIMPES (see next page).

It is dangerous to simply look at the map—or triage algorithm—and pick a neighborhood, deciding this is where I want to be. Within a safe time, the clinician must zoom in and start narrowing the field of possible disease states causing the symptoms that lead the soldier to this clinical encounter. As the clinician zooms in and gets more specific detail, the symptoms and signs become more specific. The medic threw out the GUNS on the red screen. Now the clinician can be certain enough that he is not immediately dangerous in the clinic. But what about his state of mind? The mnemonic ACT MYSELF screens for the high profile of future dangerousness, but then SOAP disciplines the clinician to examine sensorium. Is he oriented to time, person, and place? The diabetic who walked over from the ER was disoriented. Therefore, stop there. This is an emergency until proven otherwise.

Mental status changes are trapped by the mnemonic, SOAP, where "S" equals sensorium, for which the diabetic in the behavioral health clinic failed; "O" is for output, whether physical or behavioral.

It can be too much, as in mania. Did Dr. Jorden ever show that at Joint Base Lewis-McChord? Did Oak Creek Sikh temple shooter Wade Page ever show that when amped up at Fort Brag? Or is it disorganized, without coordination? Did Staff Sergeant Bales have a normal tandem gait when stepping toe-heel-toe-heel? Would that not be important to know for his fitness-for-duty exam, deploying him to a remote outpost requiring normal agility?

"A" is for Apperception: Is this soldier paranoid? How is his perception? Was Oak Creek shooter Wade Page, chaptered out of Army psy ops, clinically paranoid when he goose-stepped on

Throw out the **WWHHHIMPES!**

Barbituate **W**ithdrawal
Wernickes
Hypoglycemia
Hypoxia
Hypertensive Encephalopathy
Iintracerebral Bleed
Meningitis
Poisoning
Encephalitis
Status Epilepticus
Clear Emergency Altered Conciousness

"ACT MYSELF"

- A = Anxiety and Agitation
- C = The Combative Patient
- T = The Threatening Patient
- MY = Male, Young
- S = Strange Behavior
- E = Empathy
- L = Limits
- F = Fighting

"SOAP"

- S = Sensorium
- O = Output
- A = Apperception
- P = Psychosis

German Street? Was Wade Page paranoid, or did he develop racist beliefs when deployed to Germany during the war against Serbia? What about Drs. Jorden and Hasan? How was their perception? Did Imam Al-Awaki make Hasan paranoid? He all but said so. It appears that Hasan's "A" was not within normal range for a soldier to deploy, in that the enemy to him was quite clearly his own troops, whom he carefully selected at the preparedness center for execution while trying to spare non-military personnel.

P is for psychosis: Were any of the cases presented here psychotic at the time of fitness-for-duty exam, prior to either deployment or chaptering out for disciplinary reasons? It certainly seems that when his neighbor, a psychiatric nurse, saw inside the mind of a suicidal mass murderer that Wade Page was psychotic just prior to the temple massacre in Oak Creek, although he may not have presented as such in the military. Hasan was behaving strangely. Was he psychotic? At trial, this information may come out, because there are psychiatric records on him, whether as a patient or a trainee under supervision by psychiatrists.

It is now time for screening for suicidality. Mnemonics are necessary in practice, and can be a key element of computerized clinical decision support of triaging and working up unknown patients, most of the patients in high-volume military and civilian practices alike. Here is the mnemonic embedded from the JAL Triage Algorithm for Suicide Screening from The Digital Clinician® (used with permission):

Medical: Does the soldier have a medical/surgical illness? Many with repeated deployments have significant pain syndromes from premature arthritic conditions in their back and joints. Such disability at a young age is a risk factor for suicide because of unrelenting and unmanageable pain, and it is the likely cause of the logarithmic rate of increase of suicide rate in white males with age. Neither women nor other races show such a straight line up that correlates with age. White men do not tolerate the aging process as well as other groups of people, and young men of all races are likely the same in coping with progressive debilitation. Traumatic Brain Injuries also fit into this category and are a risk factor for soldier's suicides. Robert Bales had serious, debilitating medical and surgical diseases, including post-concussion syndrome from Traumatic Brain Injury and partial amputation of his foot. His medical surgical fitness-for-duty profile was bad enough to require a waiver from the base commander for deployment. Many soldiers with severe pain problems want to go back to contribute their experience to buddies, new guys, or their "unit" and its "patch" and subordinates, if he is higher in rank. Likely there are soldiers with TBIs who want to deploy again, too, but Bales did not.

Attempts: The best predictors of harm to self or others are previous suicide attempts or assaults, respectively.

Support: There is no better inoculation against suicide in soldiers than the loving support of his/her buddies in the unit and a sincerely concerned and respected leader, whether EM or officer. When a master sergeant comes to the ER and offers to keep a suicidal watch on an at-risk soldier by having a buddy watch suicide vigil, this is safer than hospitalization in the long term. It is like an inoculation of really caring support. This is the real solution to suicide threats in the military, but such leadership and unit morale is not always there to be called on in emergencies, particularly when units turnover fast, along with command, due to tempo of deployments and scarcity of experienced military personnel. When leadership from a trusted NCO is present, it is the psychiatrist on call who can go back to sleep for that night on call. The same goes for families and friends, whether in civilian or military practice, but good leaders and strong units are easier to judge on a military base than are families. Bales was experienced and was sent to a remote site to provide support for Special Forces Operations, despite questionable fitness-for-duty profile. Where was the support there?

Triad: This stands for the triad of arson, bed-wetting, and cruelty to animals. When all three are present during adolescence, this triad predicts homicide in three out of four delinquents. It is a warning sign of an emerging dangerous psycopath who can become a habitual criminal. Ultimately, the subject can, and usually does, become homicidal, potentially winding up committing a felony murder. More generically, the presence of this triad disciplines the clinician to think genetically, because the human genome does not always appear to connect the dots the way it would seem to be obvious. There is no reason clinically to expect that this triad of arson, bed-wetting and cruelty to animals should predict anything, but it does. The triad is the phenotype, manifesting a likely genetic abnormality still not discoverable through the personalized medicine of genetic testing to predict outcomes with or without treatment. This triad, fortunately rare, informs us that the phenotype does not easily reveal the mysteries of a person's genome. But progress is moving fast, and here is a phenotype that will yield great wealth in understanding "unremitting states of human destructiveness."

Interviews with some veterans, even some from World War II, have revealed that the psychopath can make it far in war. He can destroy the enemy with no hesitation, he can win battles, but he can also lose wars. World War II veteran of battles on Tarawa and Iwo Jima Joe Fisher, now deceased, has said that some of his greatest thrills came when machine-gunning Japanese soldiers. It was more than war; it was a form of expiation. Vietnam War veteran Arthur Shawcross, the Genesse River Cannibal Killer, now in prison, said that killing Viet Cong and watching their bodies explode from M-16 rounds was a thrill. He killed without remorse. When he returned home, he became a child-killer and ultimately a prostitute-killer in the suburbs of Rochester, New York. Both veterans talked about their childhood joy of torturing small animals and their fascination with fire-starting. Colonel Franklin Jones stated at the International Congress of Psychiatry in Vienna that Lieutenant Calley was a psychopath and the main cause of the massacre at My Lai. Two examples of serial killers and one mass murderer. Looking at this comparison, most criminologists will tell you that there is a great difference between long-term control-type serial killers and suicidal mass murderers. Most criminologists, however, are wrong.

There is a genetic basis to impulsivity in that fathers with well-diagnosed antisocial personalities breed males who are likely to be antisocial personalities, too, although their biological daughters more likely have a hypochondriacal disorder called Briquette's syndrome, with multiple physical symptoms that have no medical or surgical findings to support any disease process. Again, the human genome does not connect the dots as we would logically expect. Why, one might ask, aren't the daughters antisocial, too? With rare exceptions, such as suicidal mass killer Laurie Dann in Illinois, they tend not to be, even though they grow up with severe and continuous antisocial behaviors from their father and male siblings.

Similarly, Huntington's chorea is a genetic disease promising inevitable neurological deterioration in children inheriting the dominant gene; a 50/50 chance of such inheritance. Although the neurological deterioration seems adequate to explain the extremely high rates of suicide in the Huntington's patient, other neurological diseases are as debilitating without the same suicide rates, specifically Lou Gehrig's disease. Thus, suicidality in Huntington's seems to be associated with a suicide gene, or a genetic vulnerability attached to the dominant gene transmitting the disease. Similarly, a family history of suicide in blood relatives raises the level of likelihood for Bipolar Disorder with higher risk of suicide. Importantly, military suicidologist Dr. Elspeth Ritchie finds both personality disorders and manic depressive diseases at such low rates in military populations compared to civilian controls, that this is not as highly predictive a factor for suicides in the military.

Affect: This is the emotional appearance of the patient, and it can be:

1. Depressed;
2. Hyped;
3. Flat;
4. Inappropriate in relationship with thoughts (i.e., smiling when describing picking up dead bodies from a bloody massacre); or
5. Constricted, concealing emotional perturbation and isolative social interactions and inimicality (i.e., hiding a secret).

In a soldier, this could be:
1. Depression;
2. Mixed state of manic depressive illness, where energy is manic, but mood is depressed;
3. Emotional numbing of PTSD;
4. Psychosis; or
5. Imminent intent on killing self, respectively.

All of these are windows into emotional states with a high risk of completing suicide.

Organization: Disorganized thinking and communication could be psychosis, dissociated states of consciousness, or a brain injury like TBI. A quick screen for puzzling cases that show two or more conscious states during a soldier's life is to ask, "Do you ever lose time—for example, you can't recall a weekend picnic or birthday party, like last weekend?" Any affirmative answer demands in-depth examination of dissociative spells occurring with PTSD.

In cases of familicidal suicides, one can see the importance of being alert to evidence of overwhelming trauma, such as transgressions that boil into psychotic delusions or episodic dissociation wherein there is more than a single persona at the patient's mental wheelhouse. In such disarming patients who might appear perfectly normal in one state of mind, wiping out one's own self is not enough. The spouse and kids must die too, possibly for their own protection from the perceived evil of delusional thinking or a dissociated alter ego state visible in the horrors of combat where exposed or a participant in atrocities. For the truly paranoid delusional, it could be an act of expiation of a collective sin. Everyone must pay for the killer's guilt. For example, medic David Stewart left everyone wondering what was he guilty of. Although inferring it would be discovered, whatever it was, he took his sense of guilt to the grave, along with his wife and children. Medics are very young and undertrained for their responsibilities; soldiers die in their arms, a recurrent event leaving deep scars of survivor guilt. Who might have Medic Stewart lost in this way?

Separation: Is a patient in the process of having an intense emotional attachment severed, whether rejection from a significant other or even separation from a unit or military itself, which became family? This is a common precipitating factor of impulsive suicides, which can be completed because these guys have guns and can fire them instantly. Take a soldier suffering from PTSD who becomes increasingly jeopardized from a breakup with his girlfriend and is now living away from the unit with which he fought. He is living alone and is traumatized by the loss of his roommates, even while his buddies from his unit were committing suicide. And Dr. Timothy Jorden was pushed over the edge by the breakup with his girlfriend, Jacqueline Wisniewski, whom he killed along with himself. Separation is often the ultimate trigger.

Alone: A person alone without any support is deadlier than a person with suicidal risk factors who is bonded with somebody. Again, family members said that Eddie Ray Routh was alone, disoriented, and acting strangely when former Navy SEAL Chris Kyle took him to the shooting range to work through his emotional issues. Routh had been trained to shoot at those he considered threats, which he automatically did, even though he was shooting at people trying to help him. Such was his delusion.

Loss: What has been lost? Buddies in combat? Loss of confidence in being able to protect buddies who were killed, survival guilt, medics who cannot save enough lives or certain lives, divorce, death of loved one, disability and loss of function, demotion, or passed over for promotion are all specific types of losses experienced in the military. Any serious loss can precipitate a suicidal crisis, and such losses are very personalized, including loss of the soldier's identity of being in control and being decent, namely narcissistic loss. Sexual trauma in the theater or at home base is a devastating loss of sexual identity, perhaps more for males homosexually assaulted than heterosexual rape, which is rare in male soldiers. And it can include ground conquered at a horrific sacrifice in blood and soul, and then lost with lost promotional and reenlistment opportunities promised. Clinicians must ask their patients the politically incorrect question these days, "How do you think things are going in Iraq and Afghanistan since you fought there?" How many believe their sacrifices were of value, and if valued, what was the value? Perhaps negative, justifying despair? But, DOD pronouncements are rarely reassuring and beg the question, "Who's running this war?"

"Both the Army and Marine Corps are working to increase their ranks by tens of thousands of troops, to 547,000 active-duty soldiers and 202,000 Marines. But newly created combat units will not be able to provide relief until about 2011," according to the DOD's projections. But we face the fiscal cliff and total reengineering of the military, back to rapid deployment capability in support of counterinsurgency operations on the ground—assuming Special Operations will continue—coinciding with the standing down of large-scale boots on the ground.

Alcohol: A soldier is more likely to eat his gun or hang himself when drunk than sober. Drugs can cause mental disorganization that deludes one into thinking that death is better than a future on earth. LSD hallucinations have been known to delude those tripping out into the sense that they can fly. This has catastrophic results.

CONSIDERED IMMEDIATE EMERGENCY	CONSIDERED VERY URGENT	CONSIDERED URGENT	RECENT ONSET OR ACUTE EXACERBATION	LOW ACUITY
RED ZONE	**ORANGE ZONE**	**YELLOW ZONE**	**GREEN ZONE**	**BLUE ZONE**
Any CASE in the RED Zone means **IMMEDIATE** Emergency!	Any CASE in the ORANGE Zone is VERY URGENT and DIAGNOSIS and TREATMENT must be completed in **10 MINUTES**!	Any CASE in the YELLOW Zone is URGENT and DIAGNOSIS and TREATMENT must be completed within **60 MINUTES** from POINT of ENTRY!	Any CASE in the GREEN Zone is STANDARD and DIAGNOSTICS with TREATMENT PLAN must be completed within **120 MINUTES** from POINT of ENTRY!	Any CASE in the GREEN Zone is chronic but must be DIAGNOSED with TREATMENT PLAN made within **240 MINUTES** from POINT of ENTRY!

The Digital Clinician® diagnostic zones. The amount of time you have to complete treatment depends on the zone.

There is no fail-safe checklist or test for detecting the suicidal patient and preventing death, but clinicians must do their very best during an epidemic, just as if the epidemic were Bird Flu. By exploring every dimension shown in the orange and yellow zones of The Digital Clinician®, the examining clinician will be assured of both detecting more actively suicidal patients and being able to sleep better when one is missed, because of investing good faith effort of trying to save the patient. Not all can be saved, but very likely far more can be saved than currently is the case. There are many tools to support one's search of suicidality, but The Digital Clinician® is a computerized clinical decision support system that is evidence-based for neuropsychiatric diagnostics, including a robust profiling of the suicidal soldier, that can easily be integrated into the analytic software development of AHLTA and VISTA.

If clinicians are going to have to document their findings on an EHR, then the EHR should have computerized clinical decision support of triaging and workup. In the workup, the clinician finds depressed mood, irritability, insomnia, and constricted emotional state. Instead of putting judgment in front of criteria-based diagnostics, as Paul Miller warns against, he enters these into "problems" during computer-assisted diagnostic interviews. But, unlike today's AHLTA, he cannot simply close out, any more than he can order a drug that drops the level of another drug without making the decision to override. So the computer-assisted analytical software asks about each problem entered. Insomnia asks him, "Nightmares?" Yes. Constricted Mood asks, "Emotional Numbing?" Yes. Irritability asks, "Hypervigilance?" Yes. So, then the computer asks, "History of Intense Combat?" Yes. The clinician must either diagnose Post-Traumatic Stress Disorder, because his patient's presentation meets all the criteria for the diagnosis, or he must override with an explanation such as, "I think patient is manic depressive and in transition to manic state with vivid dreams." But now his diagnosis is both reliable and valid, unless it is incorrect. If it is incorrect, at least he had to explain why he decided to use clinical judgment over algorithmic diagnostic rules and a knowledge base of clinical decision support.

If the Secretary of Health for the Department of Defense and the Secretary of the Department of Veterans Affairs really want to make an impact on undiagnosed or misdiagnosed PTSD or suicides, then they must start with improved diagnostics, given the strong marriage across DOD and DVA clinical enterprise to practicing off an electronic health record. And what they must demand is meaningful use. What is meaningful in a veteran's diagnostic problem list with disconnected "diagnostic entries" that inform clinicians of nothing, other than nobody knows what they are doing there? So they bring in the forensic unit to review and change the diagnoses. At least the Army saves money, even at the expense of cost-shifting many sick veterans to helpless families and scarce, inadequate community resources, such as jails, ERs, and homeless shelters.

Meaningful use empowers the electronic health record. That's been proven inside the OD. Thinking about Madigan, one has to ask, just how meaningful is meaningful use? Is it to sustain the variance, as the Surgeon General questions in the Senate inquiry into the forensic unit? Diagnostic inconsistencies were the fuel propelling the operation of that unit for years in thousands of cases taken off AHLTA. So meaningful use can be for purposes of judging disability out of the context of clinical presentation. That is scandalous and dangerous, as we have witnessed. Or meaningful use can be enhanced documentation that generates diagnostic validity informing best practices and diagnostic reliability that allows a plethora of clinicians working on the same problems in the same patient over time to be on the same page. This is the alleged goal of the Wounded Warrior Program, but is that where this program is going in its investment of valuable computer development, medical sweat, and financial capital? This interoperability of collective diagnostic decision-making and records tracking is purportedly the purpose for massive investment in the Wounded Warrior Program. It should perform or be shut down, so that the veteran's diagnoses of wounds and their treatment can be reliably tracked without loss of data, or worse, one doctor is doing something that is contraindicated of something another physician does while treating a related problem.

Instead of employing armies of computer programmers working away like bacteria to have some money to live on, the departments of Defense and Veterans Affairs should at least rely on doctors themselves to suggest ways to formulate an inter-rater reliable diagnosis, which Miller proves can be done with Computer Aided Diagnostic Interviews (CADI). Accuracy of diagnoses promise validity, as Klein asserts is necessary for selecting the right treatment to reduce mortality and morbidity in any population. But for the DVA, they are working with one of the most at-risk populations ever created in U.S. history: the returning combat veteran of our War on Terror. And thus far, it's not working out well.

The benefits of our recommendations follow:

1. Better care of all veterans, both in the military and DVA healthcare systems, as well those discharged from War on Terror and future military service.

2. Significant reduction of suicide rate, due to faster and easier access to healthcare before flat broke in wallet, mind, spirit, or all three.

3. Cost savings, although initial one-off payments to satisfy veterans' recruitment contract entitlements might be a charge against future cost savings that will fund future care of all veterans.

4. Freeing military doctors to practice their specialty: military medicine, and not insurance medicine.

5. Improving retention of clinicians.

6. Taking political pressure off the Department of Veterans Affairs to allow it to change organically to meet the needs of veterans under its care, and other missions deemed necessary by the commander-in-chief.

7. End the inequities of young men and women sent to combat. Operation Enduring Freedom should now be Homeland Security, whether here or abroad. There is as much danger in the social chasm between current all-volunteer combat vets and the society they were sent to war to protect as there was between draftees and those deferred in the Vietnam era generation.

8. Rapid, economical, and service-optimizing implementation of an electronic health record enhanced with computerized clinical decision support of workup for acute, emergency, combat workups and triaging in both high-volume clinical practice and mass casualty incidents.

9. Reduced cost for military healthcare and pensions without raising taxes to pay for restructuring.

Conclusion

Wars cost money. Wars keep costing money even after they're over, because treating the wounds of war and compensating those who are the victims of war are part of the cost of rebuilding. In one way or another, that war bill will be paid for, whether by the military, the Department of Defense, Social Security Disability, or by a state or local public health and safety net. In other words, taxpayers will pay the bill, no matter which agency or mechanism the payments are routed through. The issue confronting us is not paying the bill. It is how to pay it, and how to manage costs in such a way that the bill payments don't bankrupt us or create a class of disabled that become a constant drain on public funds. This is not an insurmountable challenge, only a political one.

We must realize that the invisibly injured we don't treat often become the visibly injured who become a drain on our public safety and public health facilities—or, worse, individuals who inflict lethal harm to themselves and to others. The rampage mass murder-suicide of Christopher Dorner inscribes that apocalyptic TV image of a burning cabin into the public consciousness for years to come. We can't pretend to be the strongest, richest, best country in the world and still create an underclass of emotionally disabled individuals wandering the streets, as if they're the collective id of our population—a dystopian subculture out of a bad 1970s science fiction movie.

Freud said that our id has the capability to destroy us. Our collective id has that same capability, as history has vividly shown. How many empires have collapsed from within, such as Rome, the Maya, and the Inca, because they fed on themselves? Our own Bible provides more than one example, and Moses's warning of the blessing and the curse lays out what the alternatives are to adhering to a moral standard or abandoning it. The collective id has devoured empires, and it can devour us. The subculture of uncared-for veterans, one million of them suffering from gradually metastasizing invisible wounds of war, are just such a collective id. "A nation that forgets its veterans will itself be forgotten," said President Calvin Coolidge.

Therefore, as the one-percenters line their pockets, graze on kobe beef carpaccio, and stuff their huge tax savings into their overseas financial shelters, our politicians on the right and the left better make sure we clean up our own damage with all deliberate speed. Time is of great essence, and our id will come back to haunt us, just like Marley's ghost, to remind us of our sins. Christmas future has come.

Index

Note: References to illustrations are marked in **bold**.